An Introduction to
Healthcare Organizational Ethics

AN INTRODUCTION TO HEALTHCARE ORGANIZATIONAL ETHICS

Robert T. Hall
West Virginia State College

OXFORD
UNIVERSITY PRESS
2000

OXFORD
UNIVERSITY PRESS

Oxford   New York
Athens   Auckland   Bangkok   Bogotá   Buenos Aires   Calcutta
Cape Town   Chennai   Dar es Salaam   Delhi   Florence   Hong Kong   Istanbul
Karachi   Kuala Lumpur   Madrid   Melbourne   Mexico City   Mumbai
Nairobi   Paris   São Paulo   Singapore   Taipei   Tokyo   Toronto   Warsaw
and associated companies in
Berlin   Ibadan

Copyright © 2000 by Oxford University Press, Inc.

Published by Oxford University Press, Inc.,
198 Madison Avenue, New York, New York, 10016
http://www.oup-usa.org
1-800-334-4249

Library of Congress Cataloging-in-Publication Data

Hall, Robert T. (Robert Tom), 1938–
An introduction to healthcare organizational ethics / Robert T. Hall.
p.   cm.   Includes bibliographical references and index.
ISBN 0-19-513560-1
1. Health maintenance organizations—Moral and ethical aspects.   I. Title.

RA413.H35 2000   362.1'04258—dc21   99-049875

9 8 7 6 5 4 3 2 1

Printed in the United States of America
on acid-free paper

Dedico este libro a Mary Kay,
quien alienta e ilumina mi vida.

Preface

This book is an attempt to address ethical questions in health care as they arise on the business or organizational level: to spell out an ethical perspective for healthcare organizations. I do this, first, by considering the nature and function of an organizational ethics perspective in healthcare and, second, by taking up many of the topics with which this field must be concerned. Far from being the last word on many of these topics, given the virtual absence of relevant literature in most cases, this is hardly the first word. It is my hope, however, that this discussion will be useful to students in health services management, healthcare professionals, and healthcare administrators who are facing these issues.

Chapter 1 begins with an analysis of ethical decision making in healthcare organizational management, including an outline of two analytical strategies that might be adopted for the development of an organizational ethics perspective. Chapter 2 addresses some of the macro questions of organizational ethics through an analysis of corporate social responsibility in for-profit and not-for-profit organizations, as well as the issue of uncompensated care. Chapters 3 to 11 take up many of the topics that healthcare organizational ethics analysis will have to address. These include aspects of patient services, marketing, managed care, program development, community relations, diversity, employee relations, regulatory compliance, and medical records. Healthcare institutions are, in fact, business organizations, with most of the problems faced by corporate management in other fields. They differ, however, in that health care holds a special place among human needs and has traditionally been addressed from an altruistic perspective. Chapter 12 offers some comments on the development of organizational ethics programs that may be of interest to administrators and to professionals who serve on clinical ethics committees—especially those who are grappling with the new standards on organizational ethics promulgated by the Joint Commission on Accreditation of Healthcare Organizations.

Many cases are included not only to illustrate points but also to direct the reader's attention to aspects of issues not previously mentioned. The cases are all either real incidents or composites drawn from similar situations that have arisen in different places. Identifying details have been changed in most cases and, of course, specific sources are not cited. References to relevant documents are included: Appendices 1 to 6 contain a few of the most important sources.

Alderson, West Virginia   R. H.
September 1999

Acknowledgments

This project would not have been possible without the help of a large number of people. I owe special thanks to Mary Kay Buchmelter, Gerry Beller, L. O'Brien Thompson, Tom Michard, John Richards, Mary Lucas, Sharon Hall, Gary Chernenko, Karen Frashier, Woody Moss, Jackie Glover, Cynthia Barnette, Bruce Foster, Robin Reynolds, Drema Pierson, James Patterson, Michael Lewis, Sean Chillag, Greg Rosencrance, Ed Welsh, Les Melton, Robert Lyman Potter, Bob Bendiksen, Mark Sheldon, Paul Schyve, Jill McDaniel, Warren Point, J.K. Lilley, Elizabeth Spangler, Lillian Morris, Fran Brooks, Denise Maillot, Chuck Lucente, Martin Kommor, Joyce Broglio, Mary Lou Lewis, Mary Hogue, Charles Covert, Warren Radtke, Jeannie Bess, Abainesh Mitiku, Ann Rinehart, Gladys Kuhn, Don Patthoff, Patricia Schafer, Jeff House, and Charlie Cohen.

Research for this book was supported by The West Virginia Humanities Council.

Acknowledgments

Contents

An Introduction to
Healthcare Organizational Ethics

INTRODUCTION: MEDICAL ETHICS AND ORGANIZATIONAL ETHICS

The field of medical ethics is relatively new, but it has already become a well-established enterprise both in university health centers and in smaller hospitals. Hospice programs, nursing homes, and home health agencies are now developing ethics committees as well (DeVries and Subedi, 1998). Issues like informed consent, the withdrawal of life-sustaining treatment, abortion, the use of experimental drugs, and the confidentiality of medical information have been discussed widely in the professional literature and the popular press. Definite progress has been made: ethics consultations are widely available to patients and physicians, state laws have been passed assuring patients the ability to issue advance directives for their care and to appoint surrogate decision makers, and the automatic use of extraordinary measures to extend life has been curbed (Jonsen, 1998). Debates continue about physician-assisted suicide, the right to care that is considered medically futile, and the obligation to care for patients who refuse to adopt healthier lifestyles, among other issues.

Along the way, there has been considerable discussion of ethical questions that extend beyond the clinical setting and into the nature of the healthcare system itself, such as whether managed care is a blessing or a curse and how it should be regulated, whether physicians ought to have financial interests in testing laboratories, or whether social justice requires universal access to medical care. Other issues are even further removed from the clinical setting, as they

3

involve human resource management, marketing, and strategic planning. These fields raise questions that are closer to business or organizational ethics than to clinical medical ethics.

I use the phrase *organizational ethics* to refer to the ethical analysis of decisions and actions taken by organizations (i.e., by organizational boards or committees) or by individuals acting as agents of organizations. Organizational ethics is thus a form of business ethics, but I prefer the term *organizational* because it has a less commercial connotation and better characterizes the public interest nature of most healthcare institutions. I shall assume, without argumentation here, that it is proper to characterize organizations as moral agents at least to the extent that decisions and actions taken on their behalf can be evaluated as ethically right or wrong (see French, 1995; Goodpaster and Matthews, 1988).

For the most part, these organizational issues seem beyond the scope of medical ethics, at least as the content of that field has been developed in the United States, and beyond the competence of most hospital clinical ethics committees that do not include people with competencies in business matters. Many people in the field of bioethics will disagree with this statement—this bifurcation of the field. To some it will seem quite apparent that ethical questions on the clinical level lead directly to organizational questions and that the two cannot be separated. To others it may appear that there is no need for a separation of interests here because the same basic ethical principles apply to both areas. So let me explain, starting with an example.

Chapter 9 deals with community relations by considering a case that arose literally in my own neighborhood. The Charleston Area Medical Center (CAMC), four blocks from my house, operates three hospitals in Charleston, West Virginia, with a combined capacity of about 900 licensed beds. It employs about 5500 people and in 1996 provided $31.8 million in uncompensated care.

In July 1996 CAMC began construction of a new medical waste incinerator at its General Division in the working-class East End of the city, a section that includes both a historical district of old homes and a lower-income area. The new incinerator was intended to consolidate medical waste disposal from the three hospitals that previously had separate incinerators. Applications for the necessary permits were submitted by CAMC, but some had not been issued even when construction began. The community response to the announcement that construction had started was immediately negative; there had been no public hearings on permits other than a Health Care Cost Review Authority "Certificate of Need" hearing two years earlier that was limited to financial considerations. Residents of the area sued in the Kanawha County Circuit Court, claiming that the required permits had not been issued, that the facility would violate state solid waste regulations, and that dangerous levels of dioxin would be emitted. Judge Robert Smith ruled that the project could go forward, however, since he considered it unlikely that public hearings would affect the outcome of the permitting process. The issue was, for a while, a public standoff.

At the suggestion of some ethics committee members, the question was brought before the CAMC Medical Ethics Advisory Group, the clinical ethics committee that normally deals with institutional policy and case consultations, of which I am a member. This was an unusual case: there was no patient, no physician, no nurses, and no family. The case was presented by some of the people in charge of waste management for the hospital who were not members of the ethics committee. It involved claims of interests and rights by people (community members) who were not on the committee. It required expertise in engineering and waste management that no one on the committee possessed to even the slightest degree. It involved community relations and legal matters of which most committee members knew little or nothing. It entailed serious financial considerations of which we were ignorant, and the problem would ultimately have to be addressed by administrators who were not on the ethics committee. According to some bioethicists healthcare administrators should not be members of ethics committees at all (Wickler, 1989).

Even though I was among those who requested that we consider this issue, I now wondered how this ethics committee would address such a problem. The members of this committee could hardly do the weeks of work that would have been necessary to investigate this problem adequately. Furthermore, given the composition of the committee (physicians, nurses, social workers, chaplains, a patient care administrator, and one outside ethicist), what credibility would our collective opinion have if we did address it? Who would believe us? Our own clinical approach, at its best, was to address ethical issues by inviting all those who were concerned with a patient's care (the patient and his or her family, physicians, nurses, etc.) to a meeting where each perspective could be heard and a resolution sought. In this ethics committee meeting we had no one who was directly involved in the matter other than the people in charge of solid waste management, who presented only their side of the case; no major administrators, who ultimately would have to deal with the matter; and no community representatives.

The issue, as it turned out, was never really taken up as an ethics committee "consultation" at all. After taking stock of the situation, I did not even suggest that the committee address the problem in the sense of conducting an investigation that would attempt to find a solution in our usual manner. This wasn't a case in which a treatment decision had to be made. It was an organizational ethics problem, an institutional matter that was clearly beyond the scope of the committee; it was discussed, but it was not addressed as though the committee had any real part to play in its resolution. In fact, the problem had been in the newspapers for close to a month, local committees had been formed, governmental bodies had conducted reviews at three levels, and hospital administrators had spent hours strategizing. The last thing anyone needed was another committee—especially one with no relevant expertise and none of the stakeholders involved. I do not mean to imply here that this clinical ethics committee was not a good one or was not doing its job. It has actually been a very good committee, in my opinion. But this was simply not the place for this type of problem to be addressed. The ethical issues surrounding the construction of the incinerator were ultimately addressed—but I will leave the rest of the story for later.

The situation would be much the same with the other organizational ethics issues that I deal with in the chapters that follow. Hospital ethics committees are not really prepared to address questions of marketing, strategic planning, billing, employee relations, diversity programs, charity care, and the like. For the most part, these problems are out of their range. Different people are involved, different expertise is required, and different interests are at stake from those normally represented on hospital ethics committees.

In 1997 two professional bioethics societies, the Society for Bioethics Consultation and the Society for Health and Human Values, adopted a joint position paper outlining the competencies necessary for clinical bioethics consultations (ASBH, 1998). The competencies included academic degrees in philosophy, theology, social work, or other relevant fields; specific training in ethical and legal issues; and skills in communication and counseling. Wouldn't one think that similarly relevant competencies would be necessary in organizational ethics? If a clinical ethics consultant should have training in counseling and communications in addition to ethics, wouldn't it be reasonable for an organizational ethics consultant to have skills in management, financial analysis, marketing, human resource management, and community relations in addition to ethical analysis?

The essential difference between clinical medical ethics, on the one hand, and healthcare organizational ethics, on the other, is one of focus. Solving medical ethics problems is a matter of patient care. The principles often said to be involved in medical ethics are values relevant to patient care: autonomy, beneficence, and so on. Even justice in this context is a question of whether resources should be used for a particular type of patient and whether this is fair to others who may need the resources or who must pay for them. If a *virtues* or a *narrative* approach to clinical ethics is adopted, the situation is the same: the focus is still on patient care.

By contrast, in healthcare organizational ethics the central questions have to do with the nature and function of the institution. They arise from consideration of the mission of the organization, its role in society, and its relationship with many people in addition to patients—employees, administrators, the community, suppliers, professionals, and other providers. The organizational perspective takes its light, so to speak, not from patient care alone, but from the total mission of the organization, including its obligations to all who are affected by its activity.

I hope that the distinction between clinical medical ethics and organizational ethics will become more evident in the analysis of specific organizational issues below. In the end, however, and without reducing the importance of the distinction between clinical ethics and organizational ethics, I do not want to insist on it too strongly. If clinical ethics and organizational ethics are indeed separate, there is nonetheless enough overlap of issues that requires these distinct perspectives to be held together. If the distinction I make is necessary at this time to allow the new field of organizational ethics to develop a perspective of its own, some measure of reunification will be necessary down the road. My point is that at this time it makes sense to develop the unique organizational perspective of business ethics that is needed to address the systemic issues of healthcare administration and to bring administrators themselves more fully into the process.

Organizational ethics can be viewed as a managerial perspective. Just as healthcare administrators need to be able to analyze managerial decisions from the perspectives of financial management, human resource management, strategic planning, organizational development, and marketing, they also need to be able to analyze managerial decisions from an ethical perspective. The ethical perspective in management is focused on the mission of the organization and the people who are affected by its activities. Just as clinical ethical analysis is an essential *skill* of medical practice, organizational ethical analysis is an essential *skill* of healthcare administration. This means that organizational ethics should find its rightful place *within* the healthcare organization, not as an outside critic. Just as clinical ethics provides healthcare professionals with perspectives that help them solve difficult problems of patient care, organizational ethics should help healthcare administrators solve some of the problems they face. The exposure of obvious wrongdoing is not the central point of organizational ethics. Hospital administrators don't need an ethics book to tell them that Medicare fraud is wrong or that an indigent woman in active labor should not be sent to a public hospital 150 miles away. They may need help in sorting out the ethical implications of the issues they face in the detailed business of management. They may need support in the form of good reasons for resisting business pressures. They may need to be reminded of the real people who have a stake in the managerial decisions they make. And, like all of us, they may need encouragement to keep their focus on the real goals of the organization when pressed by the fast pace of change in their field.

REFERENCES

ASBH (American Society for Bioethics and Humanities), 1998, *Core Competencies for Health Care Ethics Consultation*, Glenville, IL: American Society for Bioethics and Humanities.

De Vries, Raymond, and Janardan Subedi, 1998, *Bioethics and Society*, Upper Saddle River, NJ: Prentice-Hall.

French, Peter A., 1995, "Corporate Moral Agency," in W. Michael Hoffman and Robert E. Frederick, eds., *Business Ethics: Readings and Cases in Corporate Morality*, New York: McGraw-Hill.

Goodpaster, Kenneth E. and John B. Matthews, Jr., 1988, "Can a Corporation Have a Conscience?" in Tom L. Beauchamp and Norman E. Bowie, eds., *Ethical Theory and Business*, Englewood Cliffs, NJ: Prentice-Hall.

Jonsen, Albert R., 1998, *The Birth of Bioethics*, New York: Oxford University Press.

Wickler, D., 1989, "Institutional Agendas and Ethics Committees," *Hastings Center Report*, 19(5):21–23.

1

ETHICAL PERSPECTIVES

The French sociologist Emile Durkheim was one of the first modern theorists to address the ethical aspects of organizations. In a series of lectures given in 1898 but not published until long after his death, Durkheim developed the concept of a professional *ethic* as a set of rules that govern the activities of people in any given occupation (Durkheim, 1957). He believed that the rules governing professional behavior are generated by the groups that dominate the profession, and that these eventually become normative standards that, in many cases, are enacted into law. Both as legal rules and as professional standards, these norms are accompanied by sanctions. Professional ethics, according to Durkheim, is a matter of following the rules because there will be a price to pay (legally or professionally) if one does not.

Durkheim was criticized by his contemporaries for limiting ethics to rules with legal or professional sanctions and later revised his conception to take account of the motivational or ideal aspect of ethics (Hall, 1987). This other side of ethics, he told the French Philosophical Society in 1906, is the ideal we hold of what society should be like and how we ought to live. It is a goal to strive for, not just a rule to follow. Morality, then, is both stick and carrot: obligatory conduct but also a social ideal to which we are enthusiastically committed (Durkheim, 1953, 1993).

Following Durkheim's lead, I conceive organizational ethics as both rules to be followed and goals to be attained. To develop ethical awareness in organiza-

9

tions requires finding a process by which the people who make up the organization can identify guidelines and aspirational ideals to which they can feel committed (Hall, 1982). One must be conscious of the role of law and organizational policies in setting standards for organizational activity without losing sight of the motivational role of ideals. When people hold high ideals for the organizations in which they work, they tend to act differently than when they do not. These ideals are often embodied in the mission statements of healthcare organizations and can empower those who have a stake in the accomplishments of these organizations. Morality is thus a pluralistic concept; it exists in our society (as laws and professional codes), in our consciences (as values and commitments), in our minds (as rational principles), and in our hearts (as ideals and personal commitments).

There is no doubt that the current interest in organizational ethics stems from the fact that many people feel that respect for rules and ideals has been slipping away. If we can gain control of our organizations, however, the trend should not be irreversible. But organizations are highly structured today, and they are largely driven by the contingencies of their structures. Although we may well carry our morality in our minds and hearts, in our organizational lives, if it isn't on the agenda, it won't get the attention it deserves. So the task of organizational ethics is to find ways to institutionalize the establishment of principles to guide our decisions and actions, and to institutionalize the social goals to which we are committed.

WESTERN ETHICAL THOUGHT: FOUR PERSPECTIVES

There are many ways to categorize ethical theories. Philosophers disagree not only about moral principles, but also about what constitutes a justification of an ethical perspective and whether moral philosophy should focus on the consequences of human actions, individual motives, or moral principles. My purpose here is to provide a broad descriptive picture of the lines of ethical theory that constitute the major options in current Western thought. For the purposes of this discussion I categorize Western ethical thought in four major groups. I use the term *perspective* to indicate that each of these alternatives includes a number of variants and to demonstrate that no exclusive priority can be claimed for any one. Indeed, the pluralist position adopted here acknowledges the merits of each of these traditions.

Utilitarianism

Utilitarian perspectives focus on the consequences of actions. What makes an action morally acceptable or unacceptable is its effects on people. Originally, in the writings of John Stuart Mill and Jeremy Bentham, it was the happiness or satisfaction of individuals that was held to be the criterion, but more recently, the concept of benefits to individuals or the fulfillment of people's interests has been the focus. In either case, the people affected (if they are competent adults) are the ultimate judges of their own benefits, and no one who is affected can be left out of the calculation. The right action is the one among the available alternatives that maximizes benefits for the most people. Moral value, to the utilitarian, lies in balancing good consequences with harm or minimizing harm if the choice is between two or more undesirable actions.

The utilitarian perspective is often helpful in evaluating social issues related to the distribution of health care. Programs that serve major interests of many people would be given priority over those serving fewer people with less pressing needs. Thus, for example, the state of Oregon has rationed health care under Medicaid to meet those needs judged to be most pressing (of greatest benefit) to the majority of participants in the program. The major criticism of the utilitarian perspective, however, is that it might ignore individual rights in favor of collective benefits for the majority.

While utilitarian calculation shares certain characteristics with economic cost-benefit analysis, there is an important distinction: cost-benefit analysis is calculated only from the point of view of possible benefits for the corporation or person taking the action, while utilitarian analysis takes into account the consequences for all people. So while it may be financially beneficial *to a hospital* to close an emergency service, for example, utilitarian analysis would take account of the lost benefits to patients who may have no alternative service available. Cost-benefit calculations only take account of the consequences for the organization; utilitarianism must figure the costs and benefits from a universal perspective.

Some philosophers defend a version of utilitarianism that applies the utilitarian criterion to general classes of actions rather than to individual acts. They are thus inclined to argue that telling the truth and keeping promises can be considered moral rules or principles from a utilitarian perspective because following the rule will, in the long run, maximize human benefit. This version of utilitarianism, however, moves the theory toward a rational perspective from which general rules of human behavior rather than the consequences of actions become the focus of moral thought. On the other hand, if the rule utilitarian allowed modifications of the rules every time an exception was justified by its beneficial consequences, this would make it equivalent to the previous act utilitarian perspective. In any case, the perspective remains utilitarian as long as any rules are justified by their consequences.

Rationalism

A second perspective in Western ethical thought focuses on rational consistency. It is often argued, for example, that an act cannot be morally acceptable if one could not logically approve of others acting in the same way under similar circumstances. It is inconsistent and therefore irrational for a person to act one way in a certain situation and another way in a situation that is essentially the same. There are, of course, disputes about what is rational. Some people argue that it is inconsistent to oppose abortion and at the same time favor the death penalty because both involve, as they see it, the taking of human life. Others defend the consistency of these positions by pointing out that abortion involves the taking of an innocent life, while the death penalty is appropriate for those who have forfeited their right to life through their own actions. The rule against murder, they say, means that one should never kill an *innocent* person.

One immediate implication of the rational perspective in ethics is the principle of respect for persons. The most influential proponent of this perspective, Immanual Kant, held that if we act only in ways that we would approve of everyone acting, we would immediately realize that our expectation of being treated as persons with human dignity implies that we must treat others with similar respect. Always treat humanity, Kant said, whether in yourself or in others, as an end in itself, not only as a means to other ends.

This respect for persons leads to a strong concept of human rights. While each of the perspectives presented here can be expressed in terms of human rights, the rational perspective is most supportive of this notion. Recognition of people's rights is an essential aspect of respect for them as persons. The Declaration of Independence makes a direct appeal to this tradition when it insists that it is a self-evident (i.e., rational) truth that all people are created equal and thus are entitled to life and liberty. The U.S. Constitution added the right to own property as a basic human right along with freedom of speech and the right to a trial by jury. In medical ethics, the right to self-determination with respect to medical care is often held to be a basic principle, as is the right to refuse to take actions contrary to one's own conscientious beliefs.

The rational tradition in ethics can also lead to some serious problems. If a person has a right to life, for example, does this mean that society has a duty to preserve his life, regardless of the social costs and regardless of his own risky behavior? Does a habitual smoker have the right to unlimited health care? Does an unreformed alcoholic have the right to a liver transplant? Insistence on rights can lead to demands that society cannot fulfill or can fulfill only at a cost that would deprive others of greater benefits. This inconsistency between the rational insistence on individual rights and the utilitarian principle of maximizing social benefits has led to numerous ethical disputes.

Still, in its many forms and with many implications, the tradition of rational consistency has been a powerful motive in Western ethical thought. The golden rule is a rational principle: do unto others as you would have them do unto you. Societies have embodied this tradition in laws protecting individuals and in laws requiring fair and equal treatment. It is simply inconsistent to treat people differently because of their gender, race, religion, age, or other factors that are irrelevant to the actions in question.

A popular variant on the theme of rational consistency is the contract perspective in ethics. Recognizing that some societies aim to establish human rights that apply to all people, philosophers have argued that morality can be thought to arise from the agreements that rational people would make if they were forming an ideal society. The requirements of such an ideal society are then used to judge the moral acceptability of current social institutions. Along these lines, it has been argued that since health care is a basic human need, people would agree that it should be universally available in any society that considers itself just.

Virtues and Ideals

A third type of ethical theory in Western thought includes perspectives that are based even more explicitly on the concept of an ideal society. I include here both religious perspectives that draw their model of the good life from various faith traditions and secular perspectives based on historical precedent or visionary ideals of the good society. The common feature of these perspectives is that they refer to some model of the good society or the virtuous person as the standard for moral decisions.

Religious idealists generally believe that the good Society is revealed in scripture and tradition and is embodied in the ongoing life of the religious community. Believers who hold that the pattern of the good life is specifically laid out in religious teachings or commandments often characterize themselves as fundamentalists. Members of other faith communities find moral guidance in teachings embodying general principles that must be interpreted and applied historically as social conditions change. These more liberal religious bodies thus often appoint committees to discuss controversial issues and allow more freedom of choice to members.

The secular version of this ethical idealism is often held to be based on the cultivation of a virtuous character. Character traits that lead to the good life include prudence, honesty, courage, temperance, and loyalty. These characteristics have been valued throughout history as essential to social life and indicative of human fulfillment. They can be developed through a consistent education that takes account of social duties and builds trust and respect between people. The ethical life, according to this perspective, is more than just following a set of rules or seeking beneficial outcomes; it is a matter of fulfilling ideals. For this perspective it is the virtuous character of the person taking the action that counts ethically, not rules or consequences.

Contextual Perspectives

This final category of Western ethical perspectives includes theories that focus on the existing social context of moral decisions. Moral duties and obligations, according to this perspective, arise out of the roles and relationships people develop and cannot be determined by abstract calculations of consequences, application of universal rules, or conformity to conceptual ideals. The problem with these formalistic approaches is that they do not take account of the experiences of individuals in their unique historical context. Moral decisions cannot be separated from the actual situations in which people make them or from the network of relationships that makes up society. People acquire duties and obligations because of the personal roles and relationships they have as parents, marriage partners, sisters, brothers, and children. They acquire other roles when they enter into business and social relations. These relationships cannot be reduced to an abstract set of duties or principles without seriously distorting their nature. According to the contextual perspectives, individuals can only know their obligations from within the pattern of relationships that constitutes their lives. Morality is thus a matter of paying close attention to the details of life and accepting responsibility for the lives of others.

One variant of the contextual perspective—feminist ethics—is especially important today. Feminist philosophers have advanced the claim that traditional Western morality has excluded the moral experience of women. While the typical Western male perspective focuses on rights and obligations, the feminist approach centers on caring for others in a network of trusting personal relationships. The question of seniority in occupational advancement provides a good example. While the organization may focus on the skills and abilities required for a particular job and attempt to use an impartial selection procedure, the feminist would try to assist existing employees to develop the necessary talents and would try to build organizational loyalty by recognizing past contributions. Enhancing existing relationships, in this view, may outweigh the value of specific job qualifications (see Chapter 10). The feminist perspective thus attempts to build on what exists rather than to recalculate or reconstruct social reality. The obligations involved in existing relationships can thus outweigh the impartiality of the traditional approach based on justice and equality of opportunity. From this perspective, the details of the situation are more important than the principles that might be applied to it; and since every situation presents a new configuration of details, decisions cannot be made in the abstract. The feminist ethic is contextual and case centered: relationships are more important than institutional obligations. The willingness of a social worker to bend the institutional rules to make arrangements for a particular patient captures the flexibility that feminists see as essential to morality.

To illustrate these four ethical perspectives, imagine that a hospital administrator receives a call from a newspaper reporter asking about an outbreak of hepatitis A in the general medical division of the hospital. The hospital has already taken quick action to contain and control the infection, and the administrator believes that these measures have been successful. Should she admit the problem and explain the situation, deny the problem and hope that it will not be reported, or refuse to talk to the reporter about it? From the perspective of rational principles, it would seem that she should be open and honest about the problem. From a utilitarian perspective, she might worry about causing unnecessary fears among patients and undermining the public reputation of the hospital. From an idealist perspective, she might consider the essential relationship of trust the organization has with its patients and their families and realize that trust is ultimately based on honesty. Contextual considerations would take note of the major participants in the situation and perhaps whether the newspaper is likely to be sympathetic or antagonistic. Each perspective focuses on different elements of the problem, and all are important considerations.

ETHICS IN A PLURALISTIC SOCIETY

In addition to the ethical perspectives common in Western culture, there is also a general background of social or cultural norms in any society. At the weak end of the scale, these norms are merely customary habits such as introducing people and shaking hands. At the strong end of the spectrum, societies develop their more serious norms into laws and punish nonconformity. While these social norms often embody judgments to which ethical analysis would also lead, the existing norms of behavior in any society do not themselves constitute a basic ethical theory or perspective. Even when social norms are enacted as laws, it is always possible to criticize the laws themselves from one ethical perspective or another.

In the past, philosophers often believed that in order to justify ethical decisions, one had to construct a defense of one's position relying on a single theory that would generate the right answers to specific problems. As a practical matter, however, while many people are inclined to support one of these perspectives more than the others, each perspective has a certain currency in Western thought. Many of us, in fact, use elements of various perspectives at different times. This may make us eclectic or even inconsistent from a philosophical point of view, but it is nonetheless the way we live and it may, in the end, not be entirely irrational to be aware of the difficulties, of the various perspectives and still to recognize that they each have something to offer.

In developing an approach to the ethical analysis of decision making in healthcare organizations, moreover, it is necessary to take each of these perspectives into account. Whether we are "pluralistic" in our own ethical perspectives or not, we now live in a pluralistic society, and we have to come to grips with the ethical perspectives of a wide variety of people. My strategy in this book is to address issues like this as they appear in the context of healthcare organizational decision making and to attempt to provide some practical analytical methods for addressing them. I will leave the broader philosophical and cultural considerations in the background, therefore, and begin at a point closer to the practical side of ethical analysis, assuming that the context is a pluralistic society in which various perspectives are at play.

This pluralistic approach means that one would not expect all participants in managerial decision making at any given healthcare organization to agree on a single ethical perspective. While some of us may hanker after bygone ages of social or religious consensus, the reality of modern society is that most social organizations encompass a diverse group of people. Attempting to develop consensus on a basic ethical perspective is not only unrealistic, it can coerce individuals and it can even oppress cultural minorities (Phillips, 1993). Despite its inevitable uncertainty, an avowedly pluralistic model may facilitate the empowerment of groups that would otherwise be stifled or suppressed. So I adopt here and would recommend an approach to organizational ethics that is socially pluralistic enough to accommodate people with varying beliefs. As Dennis Thompson has said, "we do not have to decide the foundational questions to arrive at institutional principles" (Thompson, 1992: 208)."

ETHICAL ANALYSIS OF ORGANIZATIONAL DECISIONS

Two operational approaches to the ethical analysis of managerial decision making are especially helpful. These analytical strategies can be used together, but they involve slightly different analytical methods, so it will be helpful to consider them separately.

The Organizational Goals Approach

The first approach focuses on the development and implementation of organizational goals that are commonly expressed in institutional mission statements. Most healthcare organizations have mission statements; many have ethical codes or employee handbooks as well. Given the recent standards promulgated by the Joint Commission on Accreditation of Healthcare Organizations (JCAHO), many institutions are now in the process of developing unified mission statements and codes of conduct out of previously unrelated bits and pieces of policy and procedure statements. An ethical analysis of organizational behavior can be conceived as a means of ensuring that an appropriate mission statement is adopted, kept up to date, and put into effect. The operations of departments or divisions of the organization can be reviewed in the light of the mission statement to see if they fulfill the goals and ideals of the organization.

Standard procedures and specific problems that arise in the normal conduct of business can be brought up for discussion in light of the ultimate objectives of the institution.

This approach has much in common with the direction recently taken by the JCAHO in its publication of standards regarding organizational ethics (JCAHO, 1996). The idea here is to establish goals that truly express the intentions of the organization and then work toward these goals. Analysis of the ethical dimension of organizational programs and management practices should lead to a continual refinement of organizational goals and greater experience in the application of institutional standards. So under the organizational goals model, ethics should be conceived as a continual process of institutional development involving ethical strategic planning and implementation. This approach would work especially well for an institution with a particular religious or social mission or one dedicated to serving a particular group of patients.

The Stakeholder Analysis Approach

While the development of institutional goals in a mission statement would appear to have a lot in common with the idealist perspective in ethics, the stakeholder analysis approach has more affinity with utilitarian approaches. The idea here is that ethical analysis of organizational behavior can proceed through a systematic study of the ways in which people who have an interest in organizational decisions—stakeholders—are affected by the organization's actions. Evaluation of the consequences of organizational decisions and actions for stakeholder groups, along with consideration of the historic network of obligations and relations that the institution has developed, will show whether those decisions and actions are morally acceptable. Stakeholders here include not only patients, but also employees, suppliers, contractual professionals, the immediate community, and the general public. Stakeholder analysis is an important methodological approach in business ethics.

The major objective of this chapter is to develop these two analytical approaches in ways that will be appropriate for addressing the ethical dimensions of the organizational issues treated later. In the final sections, I add a few brief comments on two topics that commonly fall within the scope of organizational ethics: professional standards and corporate codes of conduct.

ORGANIZATIONAL GOALS AND MISSION STATEMENTS

The classic example of a corporation doing what is morally right because of commitments contained in its mission statement is one related to health care. In

1982 the Johnson & Johnson Company faced the problem of product tampering when seven people in the Chicago area died because of cyanide in Extra Strength Tylenol capsules. Johnson & Johnson's CEO, James Burke, decided quickly that the company would stand by its mission statement—a 350-word "Credo" written in 1943 and now carved in stone at the company's headquarters in New Brunswick, New Jersey. The Credo states that the "first responsibility" of the company is to the healthcare professionals and customers who use its products. This meant recalling Extra Strength Tylenol capsules from stores (at a cost of $105 million), being candid with the press and the public, and designing tamperproof packaging. "We'd committed to putting the public first," Burke said, "and everybody in the company was looking to see if we would live up to our pretensions" (O'Reilly and Lieber, 1994: 184). This turned out, of course, to be the best possible business decision from an economic perspective as well as the right thing to do from an ethical perspective. Tylenol was back on the shelves in just over a month, public confidence was restored, Johnson & Johnson became the industry leader in safe packaging, and, most important to the company, the brand name retained its market value (Boatright, 1997:17–22). It was a case of doing well by doing good: according to a 1994 article in *Fortune* magazine, Johnson & Johnson is still considered a unique company because of its organizational goals (O'Reilly and Lieber, 1994). The Tylenol case is often contrasted with the Exxon *Valdez* oil spill, in which the company appeared to spend more time and money covering up than cleaning up.

Mission statements are not always as useful as the Johnson & Johnson Credo. Some healthcare organizational mission statements (often called *vision statements, codes, values,* or *philosophies*) are so brief or general as to be all but useless for the purpose of ethical analysis:

> Mission: To improve the total health of our communities, working in partnership with the people we serve.
>
> (Camcare, 1998)

Others statements of organizational goals are quite focused and commit the organization to specific goals:

> To bring the Latest Facilities in medical technology with dedicated and quality service to the rural needy.
> To provide Affordable Health Care for middle and lower income class of the society.
> To render Free Medical Service to the poorer section of society and those serving society in other fields.
>
> (Hindu Mission Hospital, 1997)

Some statements of organizational goals are implemented effectively and serve to guide the development and operation of the organization. Other mission statements may be carefully considered and adopted, only to be set aside and neglected in practice.

The primary focus of a mission statement is usually patient care—and rightly so. But mission statements of healthcare organizations quite often contain broader commitments as well. The Management Advisory Ethical Conduct for Health Care Institutions of the American Hospital Association (AHA) notes in its first paragraph that hospitals fulfill functions of education, public health, social service, and business that reach well beyond their obvious role as providers of patient care. "These roles and functions," the AHA says, "demand that health care organizations conduct themselves in an ethical manner that emphasizes a basic community service orientation and justifies the public trust" (AHA, 1992). Thus, the Advisory continues, "each institution's leadership in making policy and decisions must take into account the needs and values of the institution, its physicians, other caregivers, and employees and those of individual patients, their families, and the community as a whole." The AHA explicitly states that a hospital has ethical responsibilities "deriving from its organizational roles as employer and business entity."

Mission Statement Principles

The organizational goals expressed in institutional mission statements are seldom unproblematic. If they are to be useful in guiding organizational decisions, statements of institutional goals need to be interpreted quite carefully. This interpretation, much like the interpretation of a national constitution by courts and legislatures, is an ongoing process of applying broad principles to new situations. Consider the following principles drawn from various healthcare organizational mission statements and what they might imply:

> Valley Baptist Medical Center is a multi-purpose community health service institution organized to perform health, religious, charitable, scientific, literary, and educational programs.
>
> (Valley Baptist Medical Center, 1997)

This statement would seem to commit the organization to a wide range of social programs in addition to direct patient care.

> As a premier academic medical center, we are devoted to educating health care professionals, patients, families, employees and the communities we serve.
>
> (Maimonides Medical Center, 1998)

Community education can be minimal or extensive. What portion of a medical center's budget would you think should be committed to public education?

> We believe in providing a fair, non-discriminatory working environment that recognizes the value of the employee and encourages personal and professional growth.
>
> (St. Mary Medical Center, 1998)

I know nothing about the practices at St. Mary Medical Center, but one might expect organizational mission statements that specify ideals related to diversity and human rights to be backed by specific programs.

> To promote the involvement of all levels of faculty and staff in the identification and solution of problems.
>
> (Louisiana State University Medical Center, 1998)

Staff relations at all levels are complicated matters; the active involvement of people throughout the institution in organizational decision-making is a very high ideal.

> [The] Family Medicine Education [Division] supports Kettering Medical Center's mission of improving the lives of people of the community by offering innovative, educational experiences for learners that promote their ability to care for patients and families through a team-oriented approach to health delivery.
>
> (Kettering Medical Center, 1998)

Again, a genuine "team oriented approach" is a high ideal. This implies an organizational culture that actually empowers nurses, social workers and other caregivers as members of the team.

> Long Beach Community Medical Center, in fulfilling its mission, is committed to utilizing innovative organizational and financial approaches to increase the accessibility of needed healthcare services to assist the medically underserved, and to provide, within available resources, indigent and charity care.
>
> (Long Beach Community Medical Center, 1997)

Most not-for-profit healthcare organizations are committed to care for the medically underserved. The extent of this commitment, described here as "within available resources," and its execution are never unproblematic.

For-profit healthcare corporations may also have goals and objectives that go beyond increasing the dividends to shareholders and the value of their stock. Consider the possible implications of the mission statement of the Tenet Healthcare Corporation in light of its for-profit status:

> Tenet will:
> Meet the needs of each and every patient, whose care is our primary purpose and mission.
> Maintain and enhance cooperative relationships with physicians to better serve the healthcare needs of our communities.

Forge strong partnerships with those who share our values.

Achieve standards of excellence which become the benchmark of industry practices.

Use innovation and creativity to identify and solve problems.

Apply quality management and leadership principles to foster continued employee development.

Treat each other, our patients and our partners with respect and dignity.

Hold integrity and honesty as our most important principles and perform at all times at the highest ethical standards.

Achieve a competitive return for our investors.

Strive for improvement day in and day out in everything we do.

(Tenet Healthcare Corporation, 1997–1999)

One would need to know a great deal about the organizational culture at Tenet hospitals to know whether these goals are carried into practice, and I don't mean to imply that they are not. One should notice, however, that these goals generally refer to services to patients rather than to the healthcare needs of communities. For-profit organizations face the problem of maintaining a commitment to nonfinancial goals in a business world focused primarily on return on investment and equity.

The Basis of Organizational Goals

We live in a pluralistic society in which healthcare organizations have emerged historically in response to a variety of social needs. The people who are motivated to respond to these needs may have very different understandings of the situation and may express their goals quite differently. The institutions that were built in the United States under federal Hill-Burton funding, for example, brought together professionals with services to offer, community leaders responding to public demands, and even contractors interested in constructing buildings. This diversity did not prevent consensus from emerging, nor should it now prevent strategic planners and governing boards from setting goals and charting courses for their institutions.

People do, of course, reflect on their goals and those of the organizations with which they are associated, and some of these reflections are tied to their basic philosophical perspectives on life. If a person's orientation comes from a specific religious tradition or if the organization for which he or she works is associated with such a tradition, this may provide the basis for a commitment to specific goals. We see this often in healthcare:

. . . In accordance with the teachings and healing of Jesus Christ, the Valley Baptist Medical Center and affiliated organizations are committed to enhance the health, wholeness, and dignity of those we serve . . . to present a positive Christian interpretation of ministry to the whole person—body, mind and spirit—through the experience of disease, injury, disability and death . . . [and] to relate to those whom we serve and employ as people of dignity and worth, regardless of race, gender, creed, or economic status. . . .

(Valley Baptist Medical Center, 1997)

Outside religious communities, there is a strong tradition in philosophy, tracing its roots back to Aristotle, that appeals to ideas of virtue or excellence to establish standards for individuals and institutions (MacIntyre, 1981; Solomon, 1992). Robert Solomon, for example, speaks of the corporation as a community engaged in certain patterns of practice based on an ideal that would presumably lead to specific organizational goals when developed in a particular institutional setting:

> The Aristotelian approach to business presupposes an ideal, an ultimate purpose, but the ideal of business in general is not, as my undergraduates so smartly insist, "to make money." It is to serve society's demands and the public good and be rewarded for doing so. This ideal in turn defines the mission of the corporation and provides the criteria according to which corporations and everyone in business can be praised or criticized.
>
> (Solomon, 1992:110)

The ideal itself, according to Solomon, is a composite of individual virtues within a communal framework.

> The concept of virtue provides the conceptual linkage between the individual and his or her society. A virtue is a pervasive trait of character that allows one to "fit into" a particular society and to excel in it. Aristotle analyzed the virtues as basic constituents of happiness, and these virtues included, we should add right away, not only such "moral" virtues as honesty but also many "nonmoral" virtues such as wittiness, generosity and loyalty.
>
> (Solomon, 1992:107)

Solomon offers an account of the various Aristotelian virtues, such as courage, temperance, truthfulness, justice, and honor, with an emphasis on the social aspects and implications of each one.

Tom Michaud, Director of the Center for Applied Ethics at Wheeling-Jesuit College, applies the traditional Aristotelian virtues directly to organizations by pointing out that institutional policies and practices can be considered virtuous if they effectively foster individual virtues. "Individual virtues are just the beginning of the ethical analysis of institutions: we have to look at whether the organizational mission is consistent with and promotes individual behavior that is virtuous" (Tom Michaud, personal communication).

Some advocates of this perspective think of the virtues as universal and eternal, that is, as based on the essential and enduring elements of human nature and social organization. Others, like Solomon (1992:196), believe that what counts as virtuous varies "from culture to culture and throughout history." This view would appear, then, to draw its ideal for organizational goals from the historical tradition of a given society and the accumulated wisdom of its culture.

Philosophically, the virtues school has its weaknesses. Based on ideals drawn from cultural tradition, historical precedent, or religious belief, the virtues perspective can become too bound to past and present moral values and social structures to permit or encourage social change. It may thus lack a critical base from which the historical moral order can itself be evaluated. Defenders point out, however, that traditions themselves are always evolving and that in any case it is up to the current directors, administrators, and members of an organization to set goals that are appropriate for their own time and place.

The Content of Mission Statements

Just what principles should the mission statement of a healthcare organization contain? There are no absolutes here, but I would direct the reader's attention to the AHA's Management Advisory Ethical Conduct for Health Care Institutions. The AHA advises its members that they should be concerned with the overall health status of their communities by offering education and health promotion programs; that they should build public confidence through disclosure of information; and that they should be fair and equitable in their treatment of employees. The Advisory is reprinted here in Appendix 1. Assistance in formulating or analyzing organizational mission statements might also be drawn from the considerations of the Woodstock Theological Center's discussion group (Woodstock, 1995). The Woodstock seminar participants developed an Ethical Framework around six principles:

- Compassion and Respect for Human Dignity
- Commitment to Professional Competence
- Commitment to a Spirit of Service
- Honesty
- Confidentiality
- Good Stewardship and Careful Administration

These points are well taken and cover a great deal of the field. The focus of the Woodstock analysis, however, is primarily professional rather than organizational in nature. The published results of this seminar are clearly directed to individual professionals (mostly physicians) who face problems in the new institutional context of healthcare delivery rather than to healthcare organizations themselves. One is left to wonder just how these individual virtues can be converted into organizational policies or how the organization can foster the development of these individual virtues.

Empirical and comparative studies of corporate codes and mission statements have been undertaken by researchers at the Ethics Resource Center (1990) and by others (Kaptein and Wempe, 1998), but I am unaware of any that focus on healthcare organizations. A brief study in which I was involved analyzed 95 healthcare organizational mission statements found on hospital Web pages. Using a list of topics drawn from a pilot study, we found the percentage of these statements mentioning each to be as follows:

Patient care	94%
Physicians	54%
Professional staff	49%
Employees	50%
Community health services	51%
Public education	46%
Minorities	26%
Charity care	27%

(Hall, 1999:132)

Beyond the major commitment to patient care, as this study shows, other goals are mentioned in surprisingly few mission statements.

Unfortunately, many healthcare organizational mission statements give the impression that they were written primarily for public relations or marketing purposes. They say, in one way or another, "we want to be the best" or "we treat our patients best." There are also a certain number of currently trendy phrases from marketing consultants, like "the first choice of our customers" or "state-of-the-art" care. These mission statements actually say little about the real organizational goals. At best, they contain general concepts that have to be made explicit when an organization faces the serious question of what it stands for. At worst, they are actually intended to say nothing—to be vague enough to cover whatever the organization may decide to do.

Of course, organizations can claim that other goals are included in their overriding aim to provide the best patient care. Unfortunately, however, it is quite possible to focus on patient services while ignoring community educational needs, underserved populations, and local economic problems or while mistreating employees, suppliers, allied health professionals, and even administrators. Healthcare organizations can even treat physicians unfairly, although most realize that the physicians who bring in the patients are their real customers, so it is in their own interest to get along well with them. The fact remains that many hospital mission statements—including many formulated by healthcare management consulting firms—are worthless. The organizational goals approach suggested here poses a real challenge. If healthcare organizations are seriously committed to a broad range of social goals, they ought to state them.

Otherwise we are left to presume that their major interest is to perpetuate the organization. Based on the considerations offered here, a model hospital mission statement might read as follows:

Model Hospital Mission Statement

It is the goal and mission of General Hospital to:

- Offer care to all without regard to race, religion, or ethnic identity and, to the extent that resources permit, irrespective of the ability to pay,
- Offer health and wellness programs and health education to the people of our service area,
- Provide the best available medical care to our patients honoring their rights to determine the course their treatment,
- Employ open and ethical business practices in our dealings with patients, professional associates, allied service providers, and business partners,
- Provide a fulfilling place of employment to our professional staff and employees including appropriate compensation, healthful working conditions, and opportunities for education and advancement,
- Use the resources provided by benefactors, foundations, and public entities as efficiently as possible in the pursuit of these goals.

Organizations can, of course, encounter serious problems in formulating mission statements that reflect their goals. One problem that has come up often recently involves hospital mergers between Roman Catholic and secular institutions as in the following case.

Case 1.1 Conflicting Organizational Goals

In 1997 plans were disclosed for the merger of three hospitals in the mid–Hudson Valley region of New York State. Two secular hospitals, Kingston Hospital and Northern Dutchess Hospital, were to merge with Benedictine Hospital of Kingston (Fein, 1997). Opposition developed when community groups such as Save Our Services, Preserve Medical Secularity, and the Ulster County Coalition for Choice and Planned Parenthood, assisted by the MergerWatch project of the Family Planning Advocates of New York State and the National Women's Law Center in Washington, D.C., objected to the curtailment of reproductive services that would have been required by the merger (Merger-Watch, 1998). According to Benedictine Hospital rules, contraceptive services, abortions, tubal ligations, and infertility services would not be permitted at the merged hospital system. Kingston Hospital was reported to have provided more than 100 abortions per year, many for poor women who would have difficulty traveling to the next closest facility that would serve their needs. The opposition groups provided information to the Federal Trade Commission that initiated an investigation of a potential monopoly that could raise prices. They were also preparing to bring their case to the State Health Department in an effort to block the merger on the grounds that services would be reduced when the three-way merger was called off in July 1998.

This situation in Kingston was the result of a problem that American society has struggled with for over a quarter of a century. It was not likely to be solved by any agreement on the issue of reproductive services. Similar situations have occurred in Manchester, New Hampshire; Enid, Oklahoma; Troy, New York; Baltimore, Maryland; and Storrs, Connecticut (Fein, 1997; Lewin, 1995; MergerWatch, 1998; Rabinovitz, 1997). The question is, just how pluralistic can an organization be and still be true to its own ideals? Calling off the merger in Kingston was undoubtedly the best solution. Neither the secular institutions nor Benedictine Hospital should have compromised their basic values.

Organizational goals, however, can conflict with the public interest. Writing in the *Journal of Law, Medicine and Ethics*, Kathleen Boozang points out that there is a public interest in maintaining health services that were previously available in a community. "The state should not indulge religious beliefs at the expense of patient care," she argues. It should "honor the community's right to basic health care services by refusing to approve merger or managed care proposals that interfere with access to those services" (Boozang, 1996:90). She also suggests that the separate incorporation of such services as a secular enterprise might be one option. The interplay of the public interest (in funding health services) and freedom of religion (in objecting to providing or paying for certain services) is a complex problem that is likely to remain controversial (see Byk, 1989; Kuhshf, 1994).

STAKEHOLDER ANALYSIS

Stakeholder analysis had its origin in discussions of organizational social performance and social responsibility in the 1970s, when academic researchers and some corporate executives began to look at the ways in which corporations addressed social and philanthropical issues (Wartick and Cochrane, 1985). The *social performance model*, as it was then called, attempted to assess corporate postures on social issues as "defensive," "accommodative," or "proactive" (Carroll, 1979). The concept of social responsibility remained somewhat elusive, however. "The fundamental problem was . . . that no definition of social responsiveness provides a framework for the systematic collection, organization, and analysis of corporate data" (Clarkson, 1995:99). The concept implies some general but vague responsibilities of business to society but offers no method of assessing just what those obligations are or how they should be fulfilled. Subsequently, the phrase *social responsibility* came to refer more to macro issues concerning the relations between corporate activities and society and less to an analytical approach for ethical analysis (some of these will be discussed in Chapter 2).

In the 1980s, the broad concept of corporate social responsibility was gradually supplemented by the notion of stakeholder analysis. Rather than trying to ask in general "What are our organizational responsibilities to society?" managers found that they could grasp the ethical dimension of their activity much better by asking "What might be the human consequences of organizational decisions and what groups of people will be affected?" The term *stakeholder*, as defined by William M. Evan and R. Edward Freeman, refers to "any group or individual who can affect or is affected by the corporation" (Evan and Freeman, 1988:100). Organizational managers generally know the various constituencies they need to deal with, and community relations professionals, whose task it is to represent the organization to the public, are more oriented to groups of people than to overarching concepts like corporate social responsibility. Stakeholder analysis has thus become not only an important theoretical orientation, but also a very practical link between theory and practice (Carroll, 1993).

While stakeholder analysis is regularly used as a model for addressing the ethical dimension of organizational decisions, the concept has also become a theory of the basic nature of the firm or corporation—one that challenges, in many respects, the economic perspective of the traditional "shareholder" and "managerial" theories (Calton, 1993).

> [T]he corporation itself can be defined as a system of primary stakeholder groups, a complex set of relationships between and among interest groups with different rights, objectives, expectations, and responsibilities. The corporation's survival and continuing success depend upon the ability of its managers to create sufficient wealth, value, or satisfaction for those who belong to each stakeholder group, so that each group continues as a part of the corporation's stakeholder system.
>
> (Clarkson, 1995:108)

Stakeholder analysis fits nicely into the pluralistic perspective on organizational ethics adopted here because it is not an ethical theory per se. Although it is perhaps more accommodating to some ethical perspectives (utilitarian and contextual) than to others (idealist or virtue), it is an analytical method that can be used by people whose ethical orientations differ widely. Stakeholder analysis is a managerial tool or strategy, not a theory or a set of values. In fact, both analytical approaches presented here, organizational goals and stakeholder analysis, are intended to be neutral with respect to the actual ethical perspectives organizational managers may have. This is not because ethical analysis itself can be value free but because I believe that organizational programs and managerial strategies ought to attempt to accommodate a variety of ethical perspectives. One practical advantage of stakeholder analysis is that one doesn't have to decide in advance, or in the abstract, what constitutes the ethical dimension of organizational behavior. For stakeholder analysis, the ethical dimension arises from the impact of organizational decisions on people rather than from ethical considerations outside the context of organizational activities.

Some researchers on business management distinguish three levels of analysis within the stakeholder model—institutional, organizational, and individual (Wood, 1991). The *institutional level* (as the term is used in this context) refers to the regulation of business activities by law; the *organizational level* refers to the corporation itself and its stakeholder groups; and the *individual level* is the application of the model to specific management decisions of organizational executives. These levels of analysis may be useful in some contexts, although I do not employ them specifically in the issue analyses offered here.

Perhaps more helpful is the distinction made by Freeman (Evans and Freeman, 1988) and others between primary and secondary stakeholders. *Primary stakeholders* are defined as groups whose continued participation is necessary to the survival of the organization. These include shareholders, employees, customers, suppliers, creditors, and governments (since regulatory compliance is necessary). *Secondary stakeholders* are those groups whose participation is not essential to the organization, although they are affected by organizational activities. Secondary stakeholders include the media, the community, and other businesses. This distinction provides a way of determining the relative weight of the various stakeholder claims. It should be noted, however, that a stakeholder group that is primary with respect to one issue may be secondary for another, so the analysis must be flexible.

A more subtle but ultimately crucial distinction among stakeholder theorists, as pointed out by Kenneth Goodpaster (1991), is the difference between those who consider stakeholder analysis to be a strategic means of increasing production or profit and those who consider it to be a normative ethical orientation. Those who hold the former perspective tend to think that stakeholders need to be taken into account in organizational decision making primarily because it will be good for shareholders. Shareholders' interests, in this view, remain the ultimate concern of the corporation. By contrast, there are those who consider the stakeholder orientation to be a more radical challenge to the traditional shareholder theory of the firm and who see the various stakeholder groups as having interests with just as much of a claim on the organization as those of its shareholders. From this perspective, the organization has ethical duties and responsibilities to a wider social constituency than its financial backers.

Not-for-profit organizations would, of course, have much in common with the stakeholder view in the second of these two senses since they have no shareholders and even have legal obligations to a broad spectrum of constituencies. Not-for-profit organizations, however, can act as for-profit corporations do if their focus is on the bottom line or operating margin rather than on their social obligations. The choice between the production and ethical perspectives in stakeholder analysis is not an either/or dichotomy, however. Business theorists often advocate a balance between the two, seeing a fiduciary obligation to shareholders within the context of ethical obligations to other stakeholders (Carroll, 1993; Goodpaster, 1991). This balanced approach, however, may also obscure some of the real issues involved in stakeholder theory (Freeman, 1994a, 1994b; Nasi, 1994) or may revert back to a shareholder theory if shareholder's interests are, in the end, allowed to override those of other stakeholders.

There is also a legal dimension to stakeholder analysis. Corporate constituency statutes, now in effect in a number of states in various forms, grant legal recognition to stakeholders by permitting corporate directors to take account of stakeholder interests (as opposed to just shareholder interests) in making organizational decisions (Orts, 1992). The New York corporate constituency statute, for example, states that "a director shall be entitled to consider . . . the effect that the corporation's actions may have . . . upon . . . current employees, . . . retired employees, . . . creditors, . . . [and] the ability of the corporation to provide . . . goods, services, employment opportunities and employment benefits and otherwise to contribute to the communities in which it does business" (New York, 1991). The concept is controversial. Eric W. Orts has noted that the American Bar Association's Committee on Corporate Laws warns not only of "opportunities for misunderstanding" and "potential for mischief," but of a threat of radical change in corporate law (Orts, 1992:17).

Applying stakeholder analysis to healthcare organizations, one would initially see patients, professional staff, administrators, employees, the community, and the governing board as primary stakeholders. Shareholders in for-profit organizations, financial institutions, and government would also be primary stakeholders, at least for certain issues. The list of secondary stakeholders is almost limitless. Most commonly involved are families, friends and clergy, media and social advocacy groups (environmentalists or minorities, for example), suppliers, home health agencies and long-term care facilities, professional associations and licensing boards, taxpayers, and labor unions. Each group, whether primary or secondary, would have its own set of interests that would have to be explored. The Patients Bill of Rights developed by the AHA in the 1970s may be viewed as representing considerations that would be relevant to patients as primary stakeholders. This document is reprinted in Appendix 2. Union contracts and various professional codes state the specific interests of other stakeholders.

It might be thought that the stakeholder approach is simply a way of listing concerns that would have to be addressed when confronting organizational decisions without providing any definitive analytical solutions. Again, however, this is an approach to ethical analysis in a pluralistic environment, not a systematic theory. Its value emerges in practice as a means of developing social solutions that are sensitive to a variety of ethical perspectives. This can be best illustrated with an example—a composite of stories I have heard from hospital administrators over the last 25 years.

Case 1.2 Rachel Greene, RN

Rachel Greene has been a nurse at Spring Hills Medical Center for 13 years and has served well in a number of positions, including head of an intensive care unit (ICU) for 2 years. After returning from a short leave to care for her mother, she has had four different temporary assignments. Her coworkers and the nurse managers on two units have noticed strong mood swings in Rachel, including, at times, what they felt was an excited or hyperactive state. Sometimes her mood seemed to change dramatically even during a shift; at times she was exceptionally pleasant, at other times argumentative and disruptive. One nurse said she heard from a friend (outside the hospital) that Rachel, who has been living alone since her mother died, was involved with a group of neighbors who had a reputation for using drugs. Her former nurse manager thought that Rachel might even be stealing controlled substances from the hospital; she and a nurse on her unit had noticed that patients seemed to be requesting more pain medication after Rachel had been on duty, and they wondered if Rachel could have been using some of the drugs herself and diluting or limiting the patients' dosages. They had, in fact, conspired with another nurse manager to watch the situation after Rachel had been reassigned to a new unit. The same pattern occurred—although there was still no real evidence of Rachel's actions. The two nurse managers then approached the Human Resource Director with the problem.

Stakeholder analysis of a problem like this does not necessarily lead to a single correct solution. It directs attention to the ethical (and other) dimensions of the issue and to the human and organizational interests that must be considered. Sometimes solutions that people can agree on emerge from this analysis; sometimes alternatives emerge and people do not agree; and sometimes the problem remains a dilemma.

In this case, one would look first at the primary stakeholders involved:

1. Patients whose care might be compromised
2. Rachel, a valued employee with a possible problem and a career at stake
3. Nurse managers who supervise Rachel and are responsible for patient care
4. Staff members who have to deal with Rachel personally
5. The hospital, which has its reputation at stake

Secondary stakeholders include:

1. Law enforcement personnel (Rachel's activity may be illegal)
2. Hospital risk management and legal counsel
3. Employees in general (employee policy and rights)
4. The hospital's insurance company
5. Top management and the governing board
6. Community and public relations professionals
7. State licensing boards

Consideration of the stakeholders involved here would then lead to some of the following organizational questions:

1. Which individuals have most at stake, and which rights or values are most important?
2. What broad social values or policies are involved? What might society expect of an organization?
3. Is consideration being given to individuals with prestige or power while the interests of the less powerful are ignored?

Finally, one might use another analytical device sometimes employed in conjunction with stakeholder analysis to address organizational strategies toward social issues (Wartick and Cochrane, 1985). This typology distinguishes the organizational response to stakeholder issues as Reactive (fight all the way), Defensive (do only what is required), Accommodative (negotiate a settlement), and Proactive (innovative initiatives) (see Clarkson, 1991). Applied to this case, one could consider the following alternatives.

1. Reactive posture: Investigate and charge Rachel with unprofessional conduct.
2. Defensive posture: Dismiss Rachel in the simplest way possible.
3. Accommodative posture: Initiate warnings and disciplinary procedures.
4. Proactive posture: Refer Rachel to the employee assistance program.

It might be noticed that in this analysis ethical issues were not separated from other organizational management considerations. This is because ethical considerations are best conceived as a dimension of managerial analysis. They emerge in the process of considering all the people (and groups) who are affected by the possible actions that can be taken to address the situation and in giving appropriate weight to their interests. The stakes involved are the interests and values of these individuals and groups. The best solution is the one that maximizes these values (utilitarian perspective), is consistent with rational principles, implements the organizations' highest values (ideal perspective), and preserves the network of personal relationships and commitments (contextual perspective). Of course, this still leaves room for moral disagreement since different alternative solutions may appear better from different perspectives. The object of the stakeholder analysis, however, is to bring out the ethical considerations involved so that organizational decision makers can take full account of them.

PROFESSIONAL STANDARDS AND CODES OF CONDUCT

In addition to the mission goals and stakeholder analysis approaches to organizational ethics, there are two other general aspects of this field that must be mentioned: professional standards and institutional codes of conduct. Some analysts have developed the professional approach into a whole theory of organizational ethics, and there are undoubtedly those who believe that organizational policies will suffice. I consider these to be perspectives that address key elements of organizational ethics but do not provide a comprehensive approach. They do, however, contribute important insights to the analysis of the issues addressed in later chapters, and I will refer to them when they are relevant.

First, various professionals who work within healthcare organizations have standards of conduct that govern them as licensed practitioners. These include physicians who practice under the Code of Medical Ethics of the American Medical Association (AMA, 1997) and nurses who are governed by the Code for Nurses of the American Nurses Association (ANA, 1985). In addition, law-yers, accountants, and engineers have licenses to practice according to the stan-dards of their professions, and many business professionals are members of professional associations that set their own standards. These codes of profes-sional practice govern individuals with special responsibilities within organiza-tions, and at times they can conflict with the needs of the organization itself or the practice of other professionals within the organization. Accountants, for example, may be forbidden to attribute a major expense to a different quarter or another fiscal year by the generally accepted standards of their profession, even though it would make reports for both periods look better and would not mis-lead anyone examining the financial statements. An engineer may require a costly construction change to meet building or safety code provisions even though the difference might be inconsequential when the work is completed. A lawyer may be required to disclose certain information to a court or to another party even though the court or the other party does not know of its existence and is unlikely to discover it. The Management Advisory on Ethical Conduct for Health Care Institutions of the AHA states that

> the policies and practices of health care institutions should respect and support the professional ethical codes and responsibilities of their employees and medical staff members and be sensitive to institutional decisions that employees might interpret as compromising their ability to provide high-quality health care.
>
> (AHA, 1992)

While these provisions are clearly intended to refer to healthcare professionals, the idea of respecting the standards of other professionals is equally important.

In this regard, it should be noted that the American College of Healthcare Executives (ACHE) has a well-developed and highly respected Code of Ethics for its members, which is reprinted in Appendix 3. This code elaborates admin-istrators' responsibilities to patients, to employees, to the community, and to the organization itself. Many of the provisions of this code will be cited in discus-sions of specific organizational issues, but one point of the ACHE code is especially relevant to organizational mission statements. The code states that healthcare executives will "uphold the values, ethics and mission of the health-care management profession" (ACHE, 1998). At first glance, it may seem re-dundant for a professional code of ethics to declare that the healthcare adminis-trator will be ethical. Ethical codes often tend to be redundant in this way, stating simply that "We will always act in an ethical manner," with little or no indication of what that manner of action might be. But if this provision of the ACHE code is interpreted to mean that healthcare administrators will pay close attention to the development of appropriate mission goals for their organiza-tions, and will work toward the implementation of those goals, the point may not be redundant after all. Ethical behavior involves devoting sufficient time to the ethical dimensions of organizational strategies and decisions. In the decisions and actions taken on behalf of healthcare organizations, the codes and standards of all professionals working within the organization need to be taken into account.

In addition to but usually separate from the goals contained in mission statements, organizations generally have codes of conduct (often called *codes of ethics*) for their employees. These are guidelines for expected behavior that are more like rules and regulations prohibiting specific behaviors. They may serve legal purposes as well. Organizational rules of this sort often cover confidential and proprietary information, gifts and gratuities, legal compliance, use of corporate property, conflicts of interest, and political activities. A code of conduct in this sense can be a significant part of an organizational ethics program, but it is important to realize the difference between a code of conduct and an organizational mission statement. Codes state rules for employees, administrators, and directors that are usually prohibitions of specific business practices. Mission statements set broad goals and objectives for the organization as a whole. The scope of ethical analysis, as envisioned in the organizational goals and stakeholder strategies outlined here, is much larger than that of the corporate code of conduct.

An organizational code of conduct can play an important role in organizational ethics. It can make some aspects of the guiding principles of an organization quite specific. It can say forcefully that certain practices are not condoned and that certain standards are expected. And it can give a needed warning to those individuals for whom explicit rules seem to be necessary. Some of the concerns discussed in the following chapters do lend themselves to formulation as rules of conduct. These are collected in a Model Organizational Code of Conduct presented in Appendix 4.

Most corporate ethics codes, for example, contain provisions on conflict of interest. Essentially this means that an organizational decision maker should not have any personal or outside interest in the outcome of business decisions for which she or he is responsible. It is the interest of the organization, not the private interest of the decision maker, that should govern organizational decisions. A conflict of interest arises, for example, if an administrator places orders for goods or services with an outside company of which she is an owner or a physician sends a patient to a nursing home in which he has a financial interest. If the company is owned by the administrator's spouse or a close relative the conflict of interest may be a little less direct, but it is still present.

Conflicts of interest can be problematic. If the vendor of goods or services is a friend or a neighbor, there may still be a conflict. But what if the vendor is not a friend or relative of the person placing the order, but a relative of his or her boss or of someone else in the organization whose favor would be useful? Or what if the healthcare organization is in a small town and the only vendor of the needed goods or services is a relative of the CEO or CFO? Principles set down in ethics codes often don't apply clearly to specific cases. In general, one can say that there is a conflict of interest whenever the decision maker has a motive for making a certain decision that is not related to the interests of the organization. Some situations, of course, may involve conflicts of interest that are so small as to be insignificant motivators. If an administrator who purchases a computer from IBM happens to own a few shares of IBM stock, he would certainly not profit enough from the deal to have his stock ownership influence the decision. But how much of an interest in a local company would constitute a significant conflict: 5 percent ownership, 10 percent, 25 percent? An interest is often a matter of degree.

Conflicts of interest are especially common with respect to the participation of governing board members in organizational decisions. Board members often have business interests outside the organization, and they are often business partners of or major donors to the organization as well. Since governing board decisions may involve major financial commitments, potential conflicts can be significant. Board members should, of course, declare any conflicts of interest they may have and abstain from voting on questions in which they have a direct interest, but this is not always the end of the matter. Should such board members even participate in discussions of projects in which they have an interest? They often have expertise in matters that other board members do not have. So even though their comments may be given extra weight because of their expertise, it would seem foolish to exclude them.

The AHA's Management Advisory on ethics is quite specific about conflicts of interest:

> Health care institutions should have written policies on conflict of interest that apply to officers, governing board members, and medical staff, as well as others who may make or influence decisions for or on behalf of the institution, including contract employees. Particular attention should be given to potential conflicts related to referral sources, vendors, competing health care services, and investments. These policies should recognize that individuals in decision-making or administrative positions often have duality of interests that may not always present conflicts. But they should provide mechanisms for identifying and addressing dualities when they do exist.

> (AHA, 1992)

Many of the professional codes of ethics mentioned above also address conflicts of interest. The ACHE code spells out some of the implications of this important concept quite effectively.

The healthcare executive shall:

    A. Conduct all personal and professional relationships in such a way that all those affected are assured that management decisions are made in the best interests of the organization and the individuals served by it;

    B. Disclose to the appropriate authority any direct or indirect financial or personal interests that pose potential or actual conflicts of interest;

    C. Accept no gifts or benefits offered with the express or implied expectation of influencing a management decision; and

    D. Inform the appropriate authority and other involved parties of potential or actual conflicts of interest related to appointments or elections to boards or committees inside or outside the healthcare executive's organization.

(ACHE, 1998)

Explicit as this provision is, it still has to be applied and interpreted in appropriate situations. How, for example, is one to tell whether a gift is intended to influence a management decision? Should there be a blanket prohibition on accepting gifts, gratuities, or favors? Or should there be a specific dollar value above which it can be presumed that the gift is given with the intention of influencing a management decision? Does this apply to gifts or donations to the organization itself or only to gifts to individuals? What expectations are attached to donations? Again, having a principle set down in a code of conduct is only part of the task of ethical analysis.

Case 1.3 Conflicts of Stakeholder Interests

In January 1998, the editors of *Hospitals and Health Networks* posed this scenario to a panel of healthcare organization administrators:

> Robin Wood Medical Center has fallen on hard times and posted large losses for three years running. It's located in a decaying neighborhood on the fringes of a sprawling city with plenty—some say far too many—hospital beds. The not-for-profit hospital is the largest employer in its area and serves pockets of elderly and poor residents, many of whom don't own or drive cars. The community leans heavily on the hospital. Among its services, Robin Wood operates adult day care and other popular geriatric programs, a regional neonatal intensive care unit, a large kidney dialysis center, community clinics, and a busy emergency room. It loses money on all of these services except the dialysis center.
>
> Managed care plans have made great inroads in the region, locking in more than 30 percent of the commercial insurance market. Because of high costs, Robin Wood has lost many of those patients. What's more, several insurers recently announced plans to launch Medicare HMOs, and the state has passed legislation that will shift Medicaid recipients to managed care. This is not good timing for a hospital struggling—and so far failing—to control its costs.
>
> Despite the poor financial picture, longtime CEO Joan Morgan has the support and confidence of Robin Wood's board of directors. Many board members have

served for 10 years or longer and know that Morgan presided over years of expansion and strong margins. At a recent meeting, the board asked her to pursue affiliations with other hospitals.

MetroCare, a large health system that owns two hospitals in the area, has floated an offer to buy Robin Wood. Morgan thinks the price may be too low. MetroCare's chairman and CEO also have made promises to Morgan, offering her a generous severance and consulting agreement if she persuades her board to approve a merger with their system. The two men have made plain a plan to close the hospital and transfer only a fraction of the staff to other sites. They've given no assurance that Robin Wood's services will be continued near the hospital's current location.

Morgan also has approached two other hospitals in the city, but they recently have entered into their own merger talks. Executives from the two facilities have told Morgan that they cannot consider deals with Robin Wood until those discussions come to a conclusion. Morgan worries that MetroCare's offer may be the only affiliation possible.

How should Morgan weigh the ethical issues concerning the hospital's survival versus the survival of its vital services? What are the ethical implications of Metro-Care's offer for the hospital versus its financial promises to Morgan? What should she do?

(Hospitals and Health Networks, 1998)

The editors of *Hospitals and Health Networks* raised one clear issue: "When does a golden parachute become a bribe?" This is the easy part. The severance pay offer created a conflict of interest to the extent that it gave Ms. Morgan a reason to act other than in the best interests of the hospital. Allen Yuspeh, senior vice-president for ethics, compliance, and corporate responsibility for Columbia/HCA Healthcare, responded directly: "Morgan's only proper action is to notify the board of a clear conflict of interest created by the offer and to disqualify herself to her board on the issue."

Yuspeh was one of a panel of healthcare administrators to whom the editors submitted this case. Many panel members raised questions about the people who had a stake in the outcome. Sister Mary Jean Ryan, CEO of the SSM Health Care System in St. Louis, noted the board's fiduciary responsibility to see that the institution continues to meet the needs of the community it serves and to continue its role in the community as an employer. James E. Dalton, Jr., CEO of Quorum Health Group in Tennessee, raised the question of the medical staff's position. "If doctors on staff are not fully engaged in Robin Wood's strategic plans," he said, "this should be corrected as soon as possible." Dalton A. Tong, of the Greater Southeast Healthcare System in Washington, D.C., said that "Morgan should consider whether her hospital's services are available at other facilities in the area and whether these facilities are accessible to members of her community." Finally, Paul B. Hofmann, former CEO of the medical centers at Stanford and Emory universities, raised the question of competing community and organizational stakeholder interests:

Balancing competing obligations is a perpetual challenge in most executive suites. Institutional survival is the top priority for most hospital CEOs today. But since Robin Wood is a not-for-profit facility, maximizing community—not organizational—benefits should take the highest priority.

(Hospitals and Health Networks, 1998)

The analytical models presented here are not mutually exclusive. In fact, some research has been done on using the stakeholder model to evaluate organizational goals and codes of conduct (Clarkson and Deck, 1993). In the discussion that follows, it will become apparent that the unique benefits of each approach can be combined in a number of ways. It should also be emphasized that the organizational goals approach and the stakeholder strategy are models for the ethical analysis of healthcare organizational decisions. They are not moral theories or ethical positions that automatically generate solutions to problems or commit one to any particular ethical perspective. In the organizational goal model, it would be entirely up to the organization to adopt the goals it sees as important and appropriate to its own mission. In the stakeholder approach, one would have to decide which interests should be treated as paramount and what value standards to use in judging them. Analytical models are not entirely neutral, of course; they may tend to shade considerations toward one ethical perspective or another. Nevertheless, in a pluralistic society, it will undoubtedly be better to work with an analytical strategy to address specific issues than to attempt to find consensus on a basic ethical perspective.

CONCLUSIONS

Western philosophical thought has produced a number of ethical perspectives, including utilitarian, rational, ideal, and contextual considerations. A pluralistic approach, however, is more appropriate to this analysis with respect both to individual thought patterns and to the social context of organizational behavior. Two analytical strategies are proposed for the development of healthcare organizational ethics: a goals analysis that focuses on mission statements of healthcare organizations and a stakeholder analysis of the many interests involved in organizational decisions. Two additional perspectives—professional standards and institutional codes of conduct—and the important concept of conflicts of interest will add further dimensions to the analysis of issues in the following chapters.

REFERENCES

ACHE (American College of Healthcare Executives), 1998, "Code of Ethics" (as amended by the Council of Regents at its annual meeting on August 22, 1995), http://www.ache.org/code.html (11/25/98).

AHA (American Hospital Association), 1992, "Ethical Conduct for Health Care Institutions," http://www.aha.org/resource/hethics.html (4/29/98).

AMA (American Medical Association), 1997, *Code of Medical Ethics*, Chicago: American Medical Association.

ANA (American Nurses Association), 1985, "Code for Nurses with Interpretation Statements," in Rena R. Gorlin, ed., 1996, *Codes of Professional Responsibility*, 3rd ed., Washington, DC: Bureau of National Affairs.

Boatright, John R., 1997, *Ethics and the Conduct of Business*, 2nd ed., Upper Saddle River, NJ: Prentice-Hall.

Boozang, Kathleen M., 1996, "Developing Public Policy for Sectarian Providers: Accommodating Religious Beliefs and Obtaining Access to Care," *Journal of Law, Medicine and Ethics*, 24:90–98.

Byk, Christian, 1989, "Donum Vitae: Civil Law and Moral Values," *Journal of Medicine and Philosophy*, 14:561–573.

Calton, Jerry M., 1993, "What Is at Stake in the Stakeholder Model?" in Dean C. Ludwig, ed., *Business and Society in a Changing World*, Lewiston, NY: The Edwin Mellen Press.

Camcare Health System, 1998, "Report Card 1997–1998" Charleston, WV: Camcare, Inc., www.camcare.com (11/21/98).

Carroll, Archie B., 1979, "A Three-Dimensional Conceptual Model of Corporate Performance," *Academy of Management Review*, 4:497–505.

———, 1993, *Business and Society: Ethics and Stakeholder Management*, Concinnati: South-Western Publishing Company.

Clarkson, Max B.E., 1991. "Defining, Evaluating and Managing Corporate Social Performance," in L.E. Preston, ed., *Research in Corporate Social Performance and Policy*, Vol. 12, Stamford, CT: JAI Press.

———, 1995, "A Stakeholder Framework for Analyzing and Evaluating Corporate Social Performance," *Academy of Management Review*, 20(1):92–118.

Clarkson, Max B.E., and M. C. Deck, 1993, "Applying the Stakeholder Management Model to the Analysis and Evaluation of Corporate Codes," in Dean C. Ludwig, ed., *Business and Society in a Changing World*, Lewiston, NY: The Edwin Mellen Press.

Durkheim, Emile, 1953, *Sociology and Philosophy*, Chicago: The Free Press.

———, 1957, *Professional Ethics and Civic Morals*, London: Routledge.

———, 1993, *Ethics and the Sociology of Morals*, Buffalo, NY: Prometheus Books.

Ethics Resource Center, 1990, *Creating a Workable Company Code of Ethics*, Washington, DC: Ethics Resource Center.

Evan, William M., and R. Edward Freeman, 1988, "A Stakeholder Theory of the Modern Corporation: Kantian Capitalism," in Tom L. Beauchamp and Norman E. Bowie, eds., *Ethical Theory and Business*, 3rd ed., Englewood Cliffs, NJ: Prentice-Hall.

Fein, Esther B., 1997, "Hospital Deals Raise Concern on Abortion," *The New York Times*, October 14, B1.

Freeman, R. Edward, 1994a, "Stakeholder Thinking: The State of the Art," in Juha Nasi, ed., *Understanding Stakeholder Thinking*, Helsinki: LSR Publications.

———, 1994b, "The Politics of Stakeholder Theory: Some Future Directions," *Business Ethics Quarterly*, 4:409.

Friedman, Milton, 1995, "The Social Responsibility of Business Is to Increase Its Profit," in W. Michael Hoffman and Robert E. Frederick, eds., *Business Ethics: Readings and Cases in Corporate Morality*, New York: McGraw-Hill.

Goodpaster, Kenneth E., 1991, "Business Ethics and Stakeholder Analysis," *Business Ethics Quarterly*, 1:53–73.

Hall, Robert T., 1982, "Emile Durkheim on Business and Professional Ethics," *Business and Professional Ethics Journal*, 2:1.

——, 1987, *Emile Durkheim: Ethics and the Sociology of Morals*, New York: Greenwood Press.

——, 1999, "Mission statements: What should yours do or say," *Medical Ethics Advisor*, 15(11):132–133.

Hindu Mission Hospital, 1997, "Mission," Chennai, India: Hindu Mission Hospital http://www.hindumissionhospital.com/ (8/6/97).

Hospitals and Health Networks, 1998, "Ethics & the CEO," *Hospitals and Health Networks* (January 20, 1998), http://www.hhnmag.com/CGI-BIN/SM40i.exe?docid=100:7397&%50assArticleId=10849 (12/7/99).

JCAHO (Joint Commission on Accreditation of Healthcare Organizations), 1996, *Comprehensive Accreditation Manual for Hospitals: The Official Handbook. Update, May, 1997*, Oakbrook Terrace, IL: Joint Commission on Accreditation of Healthcare Organizations.

Kaptein, Muel, and Johan Wempe, 1998, "Twelve Gordian Knots When Developing an Organizational Code of Ethics," *Journal of Business Ethics*, 17:853–869.

Kettering Medical Center, 1998, "Mission Statement," Dayton, OH, http://www.ketthealth.com/kmc/ (12/4/99).

Kuhshf, George, 1994, "Intolerant Tolerance," *The Journal of Medicine and Philosophy*, 19:161–181.

Lewin, Tamar, 1995, "With Rise in Health Unit Mergers, Catholic Standards Face Challenge, *The New York Times*, March 8, B7.

Long Beach Community Medical Center, 1997, "Mission Statement," Long Beach, CA, http://www.lbcommunity.com/medical/mdhosceo.html (4/29/98).

Louisiana State University Medical Center, 1998, " Mission Statement," Shreveport, LA, http://libsh.lsumc.edu/fammed/residncy/mission.html (12/4/99).

MacIntyre, 1981, *After Virtue: A Study in Moral Theory*, London: Duckworth.

Maimonides Medical Center, 1998, "Mission Statement," Brooklyn, NY, http://www.maimonidesmed.org/mmcmission/ (12/4/99).

MergerWatch, 1998, "Merger Status Report," http://www.fpaofnys.org/MergerWatch/status.html (3/17/99).

Nasi, Juha, ed., 1994, *Understanding Stakeholder Thinking*, Helsinki: LSR Publications.

New York, 1991, *N.Y. Bus. Corp. Law* §717 (b).

O'Reilly, Brian, and Ronald B. Lieber, 1994, "J & J Is on a Roll," *Fortune*, 130(13): 178–185.

Orts, E.W., 1992, "Beyond Shareholders: Interpreting Corporate Constituency Statutes," *The George Washington Law Review*, 61(1):14–135.

Phillips, Derek, 1993, *Looking Backward: A Critical Appraisal of Communitarian Thought*, Princeton, NJ: Princeton University Press.

Rabinovitz, Jonathan, 1997, "University Hospital Plan Would Exclude Abortions," *The New York, Times Metro*, July 12, :26.

Solomon, Robert C., 1992, *Ethics and Excellence: Cooperation and Integrity in Business*, New York: Oxford University Press.

St. Mary Medical Center, 1998, "St. Mary Medical Center: Our Mission," Walla Walla, WA, http://www.smmc.com/ (12/4/99).

Tenet Healthcare Corporation, 1997–1999, "Vision Statement and Tenets," Santa Barbara, CA, http://www.tenethealth.com/ (2/28/98).

Thompson, Dennis F., 1992, "Hospital Ethics," *Cambridge Quarterly of Healthcare Ethics*, 1(3):203–210.

Valley Baptist Medical Center, 1997, "Mission Statement," Harlingen, TX, http://www.vbmc.org/ (12/4/99).

Wartick, S.L., & Cochrane, P.L., 1985, "The Evolution of the Corporate Social Performance Model," *Academy of Management Review*, 4:758–769.

Wood, D., 1991, "Corporate Social Performance Revisited," *Academy of Management Review*, 16:691–718.

Woodstock (Woodstock Theological Center), 1995, *Ethical Considerations in the Business Aspects of Health Care*, Washington, DC: Georgetown University Press.

2

CHARITY CARE AND SOCIAL RESPONSIBILITY

Uncompensated care is a serious issue for most hospitals in the United States. According to the AHA, 6% of hospital expenses were for bad debt and charity care in 1997; this amounted to $18.5 billion, compared with $6 billion in 1980 (AHA, 1998). And this hardly meets the need; there is still a gap between hospital expenditures and the 15% of the population that have no health insurance. This situation is reflected, in part, in the waiting lines outside many free clinics.

The question of charity care involves consideration of the basic structure of our healthcare system. It raises issues of corporate social responsibility at the most general level of economic philosophy and public policy. This chapter begins with a discussion of corporate social responsibility, moves on to the question of for-profit and not-for-profit corporate structures, and then takes up the issue of charity care. It closes with a few remarks on the effects of hospital conversions, mergers, and joint ventures on corporate social responsibility.

CORPORATE SOCIAL RESPONSIBILITY

It is often said that corporations have social responsibilities to the communities in which they are located and to society in general. Exactly what these responsibilities are and why corporations should have them is not at all clear; nor does everyone agree that they exist. Free market enthusiasts and libertarians are inclined to deny corporate social responsibility entirely. In his classic essay on the subject, "The Social Responsibility of Business Is to Increase Its Profits," the economist Milton Friedman argued that the whole idea of corporate social responsibility is "fundamentally subversive." The corporate executive who, for example, authorizes "expenditures on reducing pollution beyond the amount that is in the best interests of the corporation or that is required by law" is spending money that rightfully belongs to the stockholders (Friedman, 1997: 57). The government, according to this perspective, is the proper institution for addressing social problems like environmental pollution; this is why corporations pay taxes (Boatright, 1997).

There are two immediate problems with this traditional free market perspective. First, there is the practical reality that market enthusiasts are inclined to object just as strongly to government social responsibility as to corporate social responsibility. Neoclassic market advocates argue that free market mechanisms will eventually distribute wealth and that charity is preferable to government mandates. These claims, however, often seem to be made not so much for the sake of increasing distributive justice as simply to deny any government role in the process.

The second objection to the classic free market philosophy is more theoretical, although not very complicated. What if the stockholders—the owners of a corporation—say that it is indeed in their interest and, in fact, part of the mission of their corporation to accept a certain amount of social responsibility? Theoretically, of course, shareholders are only interested in the return on their investment. But real people are different. Corporations do, after all, have mission statements that are drawn up and approved by trustees elected by the stockholders, and these mission statements often contain social goals. If a person invests in a corporation, this would seem to imply an acceptance of the corporate goals. In fact, people increasingly use social criteria for deciding on investment strategies (see Case 2.2 below).

The similarities between this analysis of social responsibility and the mission statement strategy for healthcare organizational ethics should be obvious. Healthcare organizations are corporations that typically set out their goals in mission statements. What those statements should contain is a matter for the trustees or directors of the organization to consider, and one would not expect a private hospital to have the same mission as a university teaching hospital or a municipal hospital. But they do typically make social commitments, and it is the task of the administrators and directors to see that the organization lives up to them.

Since the 1950s, the concept of corporate social responsibility has come to replace the classic view that the economic sector is separate from the rest of society and ought to be governed only by its own laws of supply, demand, and the pursuit of profit. Public confidence in business has decreased sharply in recent decades (Wood, 1990:123). This change reflects not only a growing distrust of business practices, but also an increase in public expectations regarding social responsibility. People now seek the assistance of businesses in addressing social problems, meeting social needs, and contributing to social causes. This expectation is ethically appropriate. Businesses are social institutions and cannot escape responsibility by claiming that they are collective enterprises rather than individuals. From the perspective of rational principles in ethics, there is a certain inconsistency in corporations claiming legal protection as persons with regard to rights but refusing to acknowledge the obligations that all people have as members of society to contribute to social welfare. When actions are taken in the name of an organization, that organization becomes an agent in a moral sense and society has a right to expect that it will act accordingly.

FOR-PROFIT HEALTHCARE ORGANIZATIONS

The social responsibility of for-profit healthcare organizations has been widely debated in the United States for a number of years (Gray, 1983, 1986). Dr. Arnold S. Relman, former editor in chief of *The New England Journal of Medicine*, has consistently argued that treating health care as an economic good will destroy the professional ethic of the basic providers and undermine the social mission of healthcare institutions. From the physician's perspective, according to Relman, there is an essential difference between commercial goods and services and the profession of medicine.

> Markets may be effective mechanisms for distributing goods and services according to consumers' desires and ability to pay, but they have no interest in consumers' needs, or in achieving universal access.
>
> (Relman, 1992:100)

As to institutions, according to Relman,

> Not-for-profit, non-public hospitals ("voluntary hospitals"), . . . forced to compete with investor-owned hospitals and a rapidly growing number of for-profit ambulatory facilities, and struggling to maintain their economic viability in the face of sharp reductions in third-party payments, . . . increasingly see themselves as beleaguered businesses, and they act accordingly. Altruistic concerns are being distorted in many voluntary hospitals by a concern for the bottom line. Management decisions are now often based more on consideration for profit than on the health needs of the community. Many voluntary hospitals seek to avoid or to limit services to the poor.
>
> (Relman, 1992:102)

Relman's argument to the effect that for-profit health care will undermine the professional responsibility of physicians is unconvincing. Physicians working in not-for-profit hospitals face roughly the same financial constraints as those working in for-profit institutions. If it is commercialism that undermines professional responsibility, furthermore, one should look at the motivations implicit in the fee-for-service system. The logical outcome of Relman's thesis is that physicians ought to be paid on a per capita basis or given a fixed salary. In any case, the issue of financial motivation undermining professionalism is now more a matter of managed care (see Chapter 4) than of working within for-profit or not-for-profit institutions.

Relman's argument that competition between investor-owned and not-for-profit hospitals threatens the altruistic spirit of the latter is more to the point. For-profit organizations can offer better services to paying customers because their resources are not stretched to cover services for those who cannot pay. Furthermore, services that are unprofitable may not be offered by for-profit hospitals at all, leaving not-for-profit hospitals to care for all who need these services (Gray, 1983; Relman and Reinhardt, 1986; Yoder, 1986). This puts serious financial pressure on public and not-for-profit institutions (Relman, 1984).

In general, however, the concept of corporate social responsibility is as relevant to investor-owned healthcare organizations as to the not-for-profits. Administrators and shareholders of for-profit hospitals often point out that they pay corporate taxes that not-for-profit hospitals do not pay, discharging their social responsibility in this way (Brock and Buchanan, 1986). This comparison is not apt, however. The proper comparison for a for-profit healthcare organization is with other for-profit corporations, few of which would now claim that paying their taxes is all that social responsibility requires. Corporate social responsibility begins after taxes are paid. This is not to say that there is a single objective standard of social responsibility that can or should be imposed on all for-profit healthcare corporations. These organizations have to decide for themselves what their social mission is and how they relate to their major stakeholders. In many respects, the social obligations of healthcare organizations are similar to those of public utilities: they are often the sole providers of necessary services in a community. The public is thus dependent on these institutions in ways in which it is not dependent on other commercial enterprises. The responsibility involved here requires serious consideration and should not be foreclosed by talk about paying taxes.

NOT-FOR-PROFIT HEALTHCARE ORGANIZATIONS

The special status of not-for-profit institutions in the United States is directly related to the notion of social responsibility. In general, the term *not-for-profit* refers to both mutual benefit and public benefit organizations promoting health, education, science, culture, art, relief for the poor, human and environmental values, social welfare, and civil rights. The basic rationale for the not-for-profit sector is both economic and social (Irish, 1997). Economically, societies often permit and encourage not-for-profit organizations by offering them tax exemption because these organizations provide certain public goods and services that the for-profit sector does not provide and do this more efficiently than government agencies. Socially, not-for-profit organizations are believed to enhance freedom of speech and association, and to foster the pluralism and toleration that are necessary to social stability (Putnam, 1993).

There is considerable truth to the claim that not-for-profit healthcare organizations now act more like for-profit corporations than like community service organizations. Amid fierce competition and financial pressures, the sense of a public mission has been slipping away in the managerial decision making that now seems necessary for survival (see Wolff, 1993). Young people now obtain graduate degrees in business administration and healthcare administration and become perfectly competent managers with little or no awareness of the public mission that originally inspired the founders of the institutions for which they work. Similarly, leaders in the private sector (bankers, lawyers, etc.) can be asked to serve on the governing boards of not-for-profit organizations with only a minimal sense of the public interest involved in the missions of the organizations they are asked to guide. In many respects, therefore, the first order of business for ethics in a not-for-profit healthcare organization must be to address the public interest nature of the mission of the organization itself—to review and enhance its sense of its own goals and ideals.

The charitable and public interest activities of a not-for-profit healthcare organization constitute a substantial part of the organization's corporate social responsibility. Not-for-profit healthcare organizations are generally exempt from federal and state corporate taxes and often from state sales tax as well. They do, of course, pay federal Social Security taxes, along with workers' compensation and unemployment taxes, as required by states. The Internal Revenue Service (IRS) and state tax agencies hold them responsible for maintaining a level of public interest activities high enough to justify their tax relief. But just as the payment of taxes should not be considered to discharge the total social responsibility of a for-profit corporation, the legally minimum level of charitable activities should not be thought to fulfill what the public might reasonably expect of a not-for-profit organization. Corporate social responsibility for not-for-profit healthcare organizations begins where maintaining the not-for-profit tax status ends. The mission of the institution and the social needs it was established to meet should determine the nature of its activities. While it is quite true that the organization will not survive if it does not have an operating margin, it may also lose its character if it ignores its mission and neglects the social needs that its founders were attempting to address.

COMMUNITY BENEFIT PROGRAMS

Most hospitals provide free care to people who cannot pay. Typically, hospitals require those who apply for free care to verify their need by submitting various proof-of-income documents. The applicant's income must be below a level set by the hospital, which is often the published *Federal Register* poverty guideline amount plus a certain percentage. Charity care policies also typically exclude coverage of certain elective procedures and optional expenses. It is certainly appropriate for organizational governing boards and administrators to review the procedures of the policy, as well as the funds allocated by the institution. It is also appropriate to attempt to judge whether the amount of money budgeted for charity care actually meets the existing needs of the community.

Not-for-profit hospitals are required to maintain a certain level of community benefit to keep their tax-free status. According to some studies (Young et al., 1997) and reports (FAHS, 1997b, 1998), for-profit institutions provide a nearly comparable amount. Debate about this issue is serious. Claims that not-for-profit hospitals "do not appear to fund charity care to a greater degree than for profits" (Brotman, 1995) are balanced by claims that the efficiency advantages of for-profits are not reflected in their charges or their voluntary community service (Marsteller et al., 1998; Relman, 1984). Others argue that the proper criterion is a comparison between the charity care provided by nonprofits with the actual amount of taxes foregone—a comparison that is not very favorable to the nonprofit sector (Wolfson and Hopes, 1994).

In the case of not-for-profit healthcare organizations, the federal tax form 990, "Return of Organization Exempt from Income Tax" (IRS, 1997a), requires the organization to state its "program service accomplishments" and to report on how income-producing activities are related to its charitable purposes. The IRS "Instructions" are brief:

> Describe program service accomplishments through measurements such as clients served, days of care, therapy sessions, or publications issued.

> Describe the activity's objective, for both this time period and the longer-term goal, if the output is intangible, such as in a research activity.

> (IRS, 1997b)

Program service accomplishments can include free screening, transportation, education, vaccination, and other community benefits, as well as direct costs for patient care. It is important to recognize, however, that while most people think of the community benefits of healthcare organizations as a matter of charity care, other services can fulfill the IRS requirement. In fact, charity care per se is not required. A 1969 IRS ruling defined the "community benefit" standard as (*1*) operating an emergency room, (2) accepting publicly insured patients, and

(3) having no shareholders (Fox and Schaeffer, 1991). Operating an emergency room now entails some charity expense, but charity care may constitute only a small part of a hospital's public obligation (Buchmueller and Feldstein, 1996).

The problem with the tax structure as a mechanism for monitoring public interest activities is that it provides the public with little or no assurance that the benefits offered by not-for-profit organizations are at all related to social needs. While a certain level of services is required and the tax returns of tax-exempt organizations are open to the public, neither the institution nor the tax commissioner may have the slightest idea of the actual community needs. Taking account of this problem, in 1994 California enacted legislation requiring community needs assessments for nonprofit hospitals (California, 1998); similar legislation had been passed in Texas a year earlier (Texas, 1998; see also Oregon Health Action Campaign, 1991). In response, the California Association of Hospitals and Health Systems advised its member organizations to review and revise their mission statements, to conduct needs assessments, and to report their accomplishments as a way of documenting fulfillment of public obligations (Buchmueller and Feldstein, 1996).

Exactly how expenses for charitable purposes are managed and controlled by healthcare organizations is an important question (Darr, 1997). There are two aspects to this issue: first, whether the programs meet actual community needs and, second, whether these needs are among the community's highest priorities. This may require research. It cannot merely be presumed that any and every service offered constitutes an efficient use of available resources. According to the utilitarian perspective, the right action is the one among the available alternatives that maximizes benefits. Healthcare organizations, however, seldom base their charity care decisions on market studies of the actual needs of their service areas. Charitable care is often a very large budget item; there is no reason why it should not be managed with as much oversight as any other part of the organization's expenses.

Case 2.1 Community Needs Assessment

John Worthy is an assistant attorney general in the Consumer Protection Division of the state attorney general's office. After being assigned to monitor the sale of a not-for-profit hospital owned by the Sisters of Saint Ambrose to a for-profit corporation, he became concerned that the state had no established policy on the public obligations of charitable organizations. It was difficult to judge how the charitable obligation of St. Ambrose Hospital could be considered to be satisfied. The hospital had high debts that, it was said, had forced the Sisters to sell. The assets were valued at $39 million and the debts totaled $37.5 million; the buyer, American Health Systems, proposed to put the difference in a charitable fund to be administered by the Sisters. Worthy was concerned that the money set aside for charitable purposes would not be used for the healthcare purposes for which it was originally intended, but would be diverted to other "good works." (The attorney general, an elected official, was concerned not to appear to be "attacking the good Sisters," as he said, but he agreed privately with Worthy's suspicion that the money would be diverted to non-health-related programs.) Worthy's second concern was whether the sale of the hospital to a for-profit corporation was, in fact, the alternative closest to "the spirit and purpose of the original trust," as state law required when charitable organizations are dissolved.

Worthy was convinced that there were genuine issues involved, but that the area was just too vague to pursue any legal remedies. One problem was that the state had no established way of evaluating the public obligations of charitable organizations. There was nothing in statutory law that addressed the issue, and the tax commissioner had used only vague federal guidelines regarding tax-exempt status.

To avoid future problems, therefore, Worthy proposed that the attorney general introduce a bill into the state legislature that would establish charity care obligations. He did not think that the state should simply promulgate its own standards for charitable organizations because these organizations could be legally established for a multitude of specific purposes. Following the lead of legislators in Texas and California, therefore, Worthy suggested that the state require not-for-profit corporations to conduct an annual community needs assessment and adopt a community benefits plan or program based on of the results of the assessment and the mission statement of the organization.

The state hospital association opposed any legislation of this sort, saying that it would impose an unnecessary burden on community hospitals and that these organizations have boards of directors that are already charged with the fiduciary responsibility of carrying out the charitable mission. Furthermore, the association argued, nonprofit organizations already submit tax reports covering their obligations to both federal and state officials. Finally, the association pointed out that the specific mission of a charitable organization can change over time and that hospitals should not be held to the mission originally stated by their founders.

The proposal raises a number of questions. What sort of community needs assessment, if required, would have helped the evaluation of the conversion of St. Ambrose Hospital? And could a community needs assessment be used to evaluate a hospital's obligation as a tax-exempt organization on a regular basis? There is little experience to draw on in this area, so healthcare organizations will have to develop appropriate assessment methods. If the mission of a not-for-profit healthcare organization to serve its community is to be taken seriously, however, the organization will have to be prepared to take appropriate steps to identify the actual needs.

CHARITY CARE

The problem of health care for needy people in the United States goes well beyond state efforts to fund Medicaid programs. Currently, over 40 million people do not qualify for Medicaid, have no health insurance, and are generally unable to pay for health care. To healthcare providers, these are the genuine charity patients because there is simply no prospect of reimbursement for their care.

In 1996 the AHA estimated that the cost of uncompensated care to hospitals was about $16 billion per year. While hospitals' efforts to control costs may limit the growth of this expense, other forces tend to expand it. Employer-provided health insurance has been declining; efforts to expand Medicaid coverage have been resisted in many states; Medicaid payments are inadequate (which means that expanding the number of people covered will not relieve financial pressures on hospitals); Hill-Burton Act obligations to provide free care have almost entirely expired; not-for-profit hospitals are being converted to for-profit or joint venture hospitals; and direct federal, state, and local subsidies for public hospitals are being reduced or eliminated. According to the Congressional Budget Office, between 1980 and 1991 total unreimbursed costs (which include direct charity care plus the difference between actual costs and payments from public sources) rose from 7% to 13% of hospital revenues (Weissman, 1996). The ethical difficulties posed by this situation, according to a recent publication by the JCAHO, are unprecedented:

> Never before in their history have healthcare organizations faced such profound external pressures on their survival, pressures which at times place the mission of the organization to serve the community in direct conflict with its financial viability. The healthcare organization may have a mission to provide care to those who need it regardless of ability to pay, yet without some source of financial support, usually third-party reimbursement, the organization cannot continue to offer both the service to the patient as well as ongoing employment to its workers.
>
> (JCAHO, 1998:67)

Unfortunately, the burden of uncompensated care is not borne equally by all hospitals. Some hospitals are located in areas where there is a greater need for free care, so they receive more requests than they can handle. Other hospitals simply avoid giving care for which they will not be reimbursed because of their dedication to making a profit or to developing revenue for new projects. While patient "dumping" is illegal (see Chapter 8), there is still a pattern of sending charity patients to hospitals with a history of providing free care, thus adding to the burden they already carry. In many cases, the charity care load actually threatens the financial stability of hospitals. It also means that people who need care may not have access to it because of their inability to travel to hospitals that will accept them.

This raises the question of whether for-profit hospitals should be legally required, along with not-for-profit institutions, to provide charity care. It can certainly be argued that for-profit organizations pay taxes for these purposes and should not, therefore, be required to do any more for public welfare than other corporations do. Given the nature of the health care sector, including the necessity of services, limited access for new providers, and the financial limitations of not-for-profit institutions, however, it may be better to consider health care to be more of a public utility than a consumer good. Corporations operating under these conditions may thus be thought to have an obligation to provide public access to goods and services that providers of other commercial products do not have. The New Jersey legislature, for example, found that because "there are many residents of the State who can not pay for needed hospital care and . . . to protect the fiscal solvency of the State's general hospitals, . . . it is necessary that all payers of health care services share in payment of uncompensated care on a Statewide basis" (New Jersey, 1987).

To avoid the excessive burden placed on public hospitals and to ensure the solvency of hospitals, some states have developed mechanisms to make sure that all hospitals share equitably in the provision of charity care. In a few states, charity care is funded out of state general revenues. Other states have created a fund that pools resources from all state hospitals and distributes the burden equally (McNamara et al., 1988). Here is a generalized model:

1. A *charity care patient* is defined in state law as a person whose income is less than 200% of the Federal Poverty Guideline and who has no insurance to cover his or her care and is not eligible for any government program. Patients whose coverage under Medicaid or any other reimbursement program runs out are also included.

2. All hospitals in the state are required to keep a record of free care given to charity care patients and to report the total amount of this care in an annual report to state authorities. Charity care must be clearly distinguished from bad debt. This is entirely consistent with the notion that hospitals ought to attempt to collect bills from people who can pay. Hospitals are not, however, likely to be able to collect much from people whose income is below 200% of the Federal Poverty Guidelines.

3. From the reports of charity care, the state calculates the aggregate amount of charity care given in the state during the previous year and determines the state charity care rate as a ratio of the amount of charity care to the total gross patient revenues of the state's acute care hospitals.

4. Hospitals whose proportion of charity care is less than the state charity care rate are required to pay the difference into the state's uncompensated care pool, and hospitals whose charity care rate is higher than the state rate receive a payment from the pool in the amount of the difference. Health insurance companies and other payers must permit the cost of charity care to be figured into the rates charged or to be added as a surcharge on contractual rate agreements.

State uncompensated care pools have a number of advantages: (*1*) they equalize the burden of charity care among the acute care general hospitals of the state so that no hospital bears a disproportionate share of the cost; (*2*) they help hospitals whose financial stability is endangered because of their response to the need for charity care; (*3*) they increase access to hospital care for the uninsured; and (4) they remove some of the disincentives to provide charity care that the current system generates. The Massachusetts Uncompensated Care Pool describes its accomplishments as follows:

> The Uncompensated Care Pool provides access to health care for low income uninsured and underinsured residents of Massachusetts by paying for free care services provided by hospitals and community health centers. It was established in 1985 and is administered by the Massachusetts Division of Health Care Finance and Policy. The Pool is funded through $215 million in assessments on hospitals' private sector charges, $100 million from a surcharge on payments from private sector payers to hospitals and ambulatory surgical centers, and a $30 million contribution from the Commonwealth of Massachusetts. Patients with family incomes under 200% of the Federal Poverty Guidelines are eligible for full free care, and those with family incomes between 200% and 400% are eligible for a partial subsidy.
>
> In 1996, the Massachusetts Uncompensated Care Pool paid for an estimated 60,000 inpatient admissions and 1.5 million outpatient visits. The most common users of the Pool are young adults ages 18–44 with incomes under 133% of the Federal Poverty Guidelines. While women are the predominant users of hospital services overall, men use the Uncompensated Care Pool to pay for inpatient services slightly more often than women. People are most likely to use the Uncompensated Care Pool to pay for treatment of heart conditions and mental health disorders. As is common in any patient population, a small portion of Pool patients uses the largest share of resources. The most costly 10% of Pool cases account for 43% of Pool expenses.
>
> (Commonwealth of Massachusetts, 1998)

The advisability of state uncompensated care pools is controversial. For-profit hospitals have claimed that it puts a burden on them that should really be borne by those not-for-profit institutions that are exempt from taxes for this purpose. Writing in the *Journal of the American Medical Association*, however, Joel Weissman drew the following conclusion:

> If we do nothing about uncompensated care, hospitals in needy communities may be forced to close or merge, and area-wide levels of indigent care could fall. Whereas the amount of service to underinsured patients may be driven by hospital location and mission, the financial burden ought to be dispersed. At present, using pools or provider assessments appears to be the most equitable, and realistic, way to spread uncompensated care costs without imposing on general tax funds.
>
> (Weissman, 1996:828)

CONVERSIONS AND JOINT VENTURES

In addition to the issue of assessing community needs discussed in Case 2.1, further questions have been raised concerning the treatment of community benefits obligations when not-for-profit healthcare organizations are sold to for-profit corporations or converted to for-profit status. Consider the following electronic news account from the Federation of American Health Systems:

TEXAS: Amarillo Votes for Universal Health Services

On May 6, 1996, voters in the Northwest Texas town of Amarillo voted 2 to 1 in favor of selling their community hospital to Universal Health Services. . . . Universal not only won critical public support that would allow much needed improvements to the Northwest Texas Healthcare System, but they were also the highest bidder. . . . The bid includes the creation of a $200 million trust fund. Details of the transaction showed [that] the hospital district also kept cash and investments totaling over $80 million and that Universal paid off debts in excess of $13 million.

Universal agreed to pay hospital related costs for indigent care provided through Northwest and its primary-care clinic. This agreement sealed the approval of Dr. J. Rush Pierce, Jr., Medical Director, Community Health Service, for the local health system. Dr. Pierce said Universal's commitment to indigent care and discussions with physicians working at other Universal hospitals won his support. . . . Without Universal's help, the Northwest Texas Healthcare System faced a difficult future. . . . Now, the Globe-News reports, "Sale of the hospital would eliminate ad valorem taxes, reducing Amarillo residents' burden by more than $8.5 million. . . . In addition, Universal would pay property taxes and other local taxes estimated at more than $3 million annually, resulting in an $11 million net gain to the community."

(FAHS, 1997b)

Conversion can happen in a number of ways: a not-for-profit can simply decide to sell stock, it can sell out to a for-profit company, or it can merge with a for-profit corporation. In any of these cases, once an individual or a for-profit corporation has ownership rights, the organization forfeits its not-for-profit status. Other conversions are more controversial: a not-for-profit corporation can transfer substantial assets to a for-profit subsidiary or it can enter into a joint venture with a for-profit corporation. In either of these cases, although the not-for-profit corporation has no owners, a case can be made that a conversion has taken place if it becomes incapable of fulfilling its charitable obligations. The IRS does require not-for-profit organizations to account for transfers of cash or other assets to other organizations that are exempt under Section 501(c) of the Tax Code, and transfers of assets to nonexempt organizations or corporations are illegal. But the range of options for corporate structures and joint ventures is wide, and assets previously devoted to charity care can easily get lost in the process.

Conversions, mergers, and joint ventures became common in the 1990s. In 1996, according to an IRS report, there were 768 hospital mergers in the United States and 48 hospitals were converted to for-profit status (Pichon, 1997). As payment mechanisms became more restrictive—with the advent of the Medicare prospective payment system (diagnosis related groups) and preferred provider contracts—economically marginal hospitals became less able to cover their bills. Because specialty hospitals have taken some of the more profitable services away from large urban hospitals, the latter institutions have been left with a greater percentage of services that operate at a loss. And as cost shifting has been reduced or eliminated, hospitals with large charity case loads have begun to operate in the red. For-profit corporations have competitive advantages. They can achieve cost savings through economies of scale in purchasing; cut or eliminate charity care; close unprofitable services such as emergency departments; and raise money for modernization programs more easily (see FAHS, 1997a, 1998).

Two questions have been raised about conversions and joint ventures (Marsteller et al., 1998). First, have assets been illegally converted to for-profit status by being transferred or undervalued when a merger or conversion takes place? Second, can the public reasonably expect a continuance of community benefits after the conversion? The first is a question about the conversion itself. When a not-for-profit hospital is sold to a for-profit company, the hospital property is assessed to determine its current value, and that amount, less any outstanding debts, is understood to be the remaining charitable obligation of the institution. These funds must be used for charitable purposes according to the original mission of the institution. In some situations, however, the property may be undervalued when it is assessed, thereby allowing assets that really should retain their not-for-profit status to be converted to for-profit use and ownership. According to the Community Health Assets Project of San Francisco,

> in 1984, Pacificare, a nonprofit HMO, was valued and sold to insiders for $360,000. One year later, on the stock market, the for-profit HMO was worth $45 million. In 1985, a physician group purchased Group Health of Greater St. Louis, a nonprofit HMO, for $4 million or $.33 cents a share, and the $4 million value of the nonprofit was dedicated to charitable purposes. One year later, a quarter of Group Health's stock sold for $10 million, or $14.28 a share. Similarly, and also in 1984, Greater Delaware Valley Health Care in Pennsylvania was valued and sold to investors for $100,000, and this amount was donated to nonprofit hospitals in the area. In 1986, the for-profit sold on the stock market for $20 million. Thus, in each of these deals, the nonprofit was undervalued and the real value of the nonprofits went to investors, not the public.
>
> (Consumers Union, 1996)

At times, public officials have taken action to challenge the legality of conversions. In 1996, Ohio Attorney General Betty Montgomery filed suit to preserve the charitable assets held by Blue Cross & Blue Shield of Ohio. "Before Blue Cross & Blue Shield can be sold to a for-profit company," she said, "the charitable assets that it holds must be fairly valued and the proceeds from the sale of those assets must go to a charitable cause" (Montgomery, 1996:1). In other situations, conversion of an institution may not be the best alternative in light of its original public mission. In December 1996, Attorney General Scott Harshbarger of Massachusetts held a public hearing to determine whether the sale of Metrowest Medical Center in Framingham to the Columbia/HCA Healthcare Corporation was "the best alternative available to the nonprofit, as required by Massachusetts charities laws" (Harshbarger, 1996:1–2). In 1997 the State of Oregon passed a law requiring the approval of the attorney general for the sale of a nonprofit hospital. The attorney general must hold a public hearing on the issue and can deny a planned conversion if it will reduce the availability of services, if the price does not reflect the fair market value, or if the proceeds will not be used in a way that is consistent with the original charitable mission (Oregon Health Action Campaign, 1991).

The second question concerns what happens to the community needs as a result of the conversion. If the needs still exist and are not being met, then the not-for-profit healthcare organization will have given up its mission and the beneficiaries will have lost their stake. There is considerable debate about the level of charity care offered by for-profit hospitals that have been converted from not-for-profit status. The picture is even more complicated with joint for- and not-for-profit ventures (Meyer, 1996). Boards of directors and administrators of not-for-profit institutions may be hard pressed to keep their organizations solvent, but abandoning their moral commitments, which is essentially what happens in a conversion, is an unacceptable solution from an ethical perspective.

In 1997 the board of trustees of the AHA approved a set of guidelines for its members who are considering proposals to change ownership or control (AHA,1999). A number of the principles stated in this document emphasize the ethical obligations of healthcare organizations. These include giving early public notice of the proposal, working with the community to identify its needs, paying attention to the compatibility of values and goals, providing fair valuation of assets, and allowing an opportunity for public comment. Excerpts from this AHA document are included in Appendix 5.

Case 2.2 Socially Responsible Investing

A relatively new ethical concern for corporations and individuals alike is the responsibility involved in investing. This affects pension funds, corporate reserves, endowments, and foundations. Consider the following case.

The Carter Foundation manages an endowment of $24 million. The proceeds of the endowment are to be used for medical education and research at Carter Memorial Hospital. The Foundation was established in 1962 by a donation from the estate of Charles W. Carter, whose grandfather had founded the hospital in 1921, and has grown over the years by the addition of other donations. It has supported the establishment of the associate degree in nursing program at Parkersburg Community College and the development of the Carter Memorial Cancer Center.

The trustees of the Foundation are now considering a proposal made by Ruth Walker, the only Carter family member now on the board of directors. Dr. Walker, a college English professor and prominent environmental activist, is concerned that the Foundation has not been making its investments wisely. The funds have been managed by Henry Long, president of the Union National Bank, who has followed a conservative strategy of placing the money in the bonds and stocks of large corporations. Dr. Walker noticed that the endowment holdings included major investments in Northeast Paper, Inc., a company recently criticized by the Nature Conservancy for dumping dioxin in the Quantaug River. After obtaining advice from the Interfaith Council for Corporate Social Responsibility and the Council on Economic Priorities, Dr. Walker proposed the following investment strategy:

1. Twenty-five percent of the endowment of the Carter Foundation should be invested in regional businesses to support the growth of the local economy.
2. Twenty-five percent of the endowment should be invested in health promotion organizations
3. Fifty percent of the endowment should be invested in corporate stocks and bonds, provided that the companies in which the money is invested have acceptable records on environmental protection, fair labor practices, and affirmative action for women and minorities. Corporations involved in nuclear power, tobacco, or alcohol products would be excluded.

Henry Long voiced serious objections to the plan. He argued that the primary responsibility of trustees of endowments is to ensure the security and growth of the funds entrusted to them. Trustees, he said, are not supposed to act on their personal beliefs or values; they are entrusted to carry out the wishes of those who established the trust. Using social or ethical criteria, which would lead to a smaller return on investments, is a misuse of their power. The responsibility of trustees, he pointed out, is established in law. The fiduciary duty is defined as obtaining the best rate of return with the least possible risk. According to Long, the investment strategy proposed by Dr. Walker would do neither.

Dr. Walker, in turn, cited studies showing that mutual funds that withdrew investments from South Africa in the early 1980s did no worse than funds that kept those investments (Domini, 1984). There are no data to indicate how well regional investments would do by comparison, she admitted, but the hospital and the Foundation have a natural interest in supporting the local economy, and this would work to their financial benefit in the long run. Furthermore, she said, it was indeed the will of those who established the fund that their money be put to the best social use; her grandfather, Charles W. Carter, would have supported her environmental interests and the other social "screens" she is proposing for the endowment. These questions need to be considered from the perspective of the Foundation's mission, its status as a nonprofit organization, and with respect to its responsibility to its stakeholders, she said. Investing in the community or the state, according to Dr. Walker, would be wise for a foundation committed to improving the health of the people in the area, from the point of view of both the long-range advantage to the hospital itself and its mission to enhance the quality of life of its community stakeholders.

"Consider this," Dr. Walker said at a trustees' meeting: "Apart from its illegality, would the Foundation want to invest in a drug ring or a prostitution chain if the trustees

knew that it would bring five times the return on the funds that they could obtain elsewhere?" Her point was that there are some investments that the trustees would not con-
done even if they were extremely profitable. "If this is so," she insisted, "the nature of all
investments ought to be open to ethical consideration, and the Foundation ought to consider its investment strategy in the light of its original purposes and goals."

In principle, socially responsible investing is a natural extension of an organizational
mission—an effort to ensure that the mission guides all organizational activities. A seminar at a recent conference of the Catholic Health Association promoted the idea of social
investing as an opportunity to educate the organization and its stakeholders and because
"it affords the Catholic healthcare ministry a powerful tool for changing society in a way
that is consistent with our values" (CHAUSA, 1999). The concept does raise a number
of questions, however. Should a healthcare organization be willing to accept a slightly
smaller return on its investments to accomplish its own purposes? Does social investing
make any difference at all, given the likelihood that other investors will purchase the
securities that the organization sells? Should a for-profit corporation adopt a socially
responsible investment strategy? (See McVeigh, 1998; GreenMoney Journal, 1995–1998;
Social Investment Forum, 1999.)

CONCLUSION

Healthcare organizations have social responsibilities that arise from their unique
position as providers of essential services. For-profit healthcare organizations
should take account of public expectations when formulating their mission statements by including appropriate social goals as well as return on shareholder
equity. Not-for-profit healthcare organizations should have missions dedicated
primarily to the public interest. This implies a commitment to not-for-profit ideals
that should override competitive market pressures. Expectations of public benefit
stated in tax law should be addressed through community needs assessment.
Primary among these benefits is the provision of charity care—a public obligation that should be shared by for-profit and not-for profit institutions. The social
responsibility of healthcare organizations should be given special consideration,
furthermore, as conversions and joint ventures are considered.

REFERENCES

AHA (American Hospital Association), 1998, "Annual Survey," Chicago: American
    Hospital Association.
——, 1999, "Community Accountability with Changes in the Ownership or Control of
    Hospitals or Health Systems," http://www.aha.org/ar/ownership.html (12/4/99).
Boatright, John R., 1997, Ethics and the Conduct of Business, 2nd ed., Upper Saddle
    River, NJ: Prentice-Hall.

Brock, Dan W., and Allen Buchanan, 1986, "Ethical Issues in For-Profit Health Care," in Bradford H. Gray, ed., *For-Profit Enterprise in Health Care*, Washington, DC: National Academy Press.

Brotman, Billie Ann, 1995, "Hospital Indigent Care Expenditures," *Journal of Health Care Finance*, 21:76–79.

Buchmueller, Thomas C., and Paul J. Feldstein, 1996, "Hospital Community Benefits Other Than Charity Care; Implications for Tax Exemption and Public Policy," *Hospital and Health Services Administration*, 41:461–472.

California, 1998, *West's Annotated California Health and Safety Codes* 127345, 127350.

CHAUSA (Catholic Health Association of the United States), 1999, "Mission-Based Investing in Catholic Healthcare," http://www.chausa.org/calendar/9902MBI.ASP (5/2/99).

Commonwealth of Massachusetts: Division of Health Care Finance and Policy, 1998, "Uncompensated Care," Boston, MA: http://www.state.ma.us/dhcfp (8/28/98).

Consumers Union/Center for Community Health Action, 1996, *The Conversion of Non-Profit Health Care Organizations into For-Profit Corporations,* San Francisco: Consumers Union—The Center for Community Health Action.

Darr, Kurt, 1997, "The Social Responsibility of Hospitals," *Hospital Topics*, 75(1):4–8.

Domini, Amy, 1984, *Ethical Investing*, Reading, MA: Addison-Wesley.

FAHS (Federation of American Health Systems), 1997a, "Understanding Hospital Conversions," http://www.fahs.com/public/publications/ (3/2/98).

——, 1997b, "Industry Overview," http://www.fahs.com/public/publications/a_report/overview.html (3/2/98).

——, 1998, "GAO Dispels Myths on Hospital Change of Ownership" (press release, January 13), Washington, DC, http://www.fahs.com/public/publications/press_re/gaostudy.html (3/2/98).

Ferrell, O. C., and John Fraedrich, 1994, *Business Ethics: Ethical Decision Making and Cases*, 2nd ed., Boston: Houghton Mifflin.

Fox, Daniel M., and Daniel C. Schaeffer, 1991, "Tax Administration as Health Policy: Hospitals, The Internal Revenue Service, and the Courts," *Journal of Health Politics, Policy and Law*, 16(2):251–279.

Friedman, Milton, 1997, "The Social Responsibility of Business Is to Increase Its Profits," in Tom L. Beauchamp, and Norman E. Bowie, eds., *Ethical Theory and Business*, 5th ed., Upper Saddle River, NJ: Prentice-Hall.

Gray, Bradford H., ed., 1983, *The New Health Care for Profit: Doctors and Hospitals in a Competitive Environment*, Washington, DC: National Academy Press.

——, ed., 1986, *For-Profit Enterprise in Health Care*, Washington, DC: National Academy Press.

GreenMoney Journal and the RCC Group, Inc., 1995–1998, "GreenMoney On-Line Guide," Spokane, WA, http://www.greenmoney.com/index.htm (12/4/99).

Harshbarger, Scott, 1996, "Attorney General's Opening Remarks" (news release attachment), Boston: Office of the Attorney General.

Herzlinger, Regina E., 1996, "Can Public Trust in Nonprofits and Governments Be Restored?" *Harvard Business Review*, 74(2):97–107.

Irish, Leon E., 1997, "The Role and Purpose of the Not-for-Profit Sector," Washington, DC: International Center for Not-for-Profit Law, http://www.icnl.org (1/16/98).

IRS (Internal Revenue Service), 1997a, "1997 Form 990, Return of Organization Exempt from Income Tax," http://www.irs.ustreas.gov/prod/forms_pubs/forms.html (12/4/99).

———, 1997b, "1997 Instructions for Form 990 and Form 990-EZ, Return of Organization Exempt from Income Tax and Short Form Return of Organization Exempt from Income Tax," http://www.irs.ustreas.gov/prod/forms_pubs/forms.html (12/4/99).

JCAHO (Joint Commission on Accreditation of Healthcare Organizations, 1998, *Ethical Issues and Patient Rights Across the Continuum of Care*, Chicago: Joint Commission on Accreditation of Healthcare Organizations.

Marsteller, Jill A., Randall R. Bovbjerg, and Len M. Nichols, 1998, "Nonprofit Conversion: Theory, Evidence and State Policy," *Health Services Research*, 33(5):1495–1498.

McNamara, Margaret C., Christine M. Grant, and Scott Crawford, 1988, "Financing Uncompensated Care Under Hospital Price Competition: New Jersey's Approach," *Trustee: The Magazine for Hospital Governing Boards*, October, 14–15.

McVeigh, Patrick, 1998, "The Best Socially Screened Mutual Funds for 1998," *Business Ethics*.

Meyer, Harris, 1996, "The Deal," *Hospital and Health Networks*, 70:36–39.

Montgomery, Betty G., 1996, "Attorney General Montgomery Intervenes in Blue Cross & Blue Shield Deal with Columbia/HCA to Protect Charitable Assets" (news release, 7/11/96), Columbus, OH: Office of the Attorney General.

New Jersey, 1987, *N.J.A.C.* 26:2H-4.1 [repealed 1991].

Oregon Health Action Campaign, 1991, "Mergers, Acquisitions and Community Benefits Task Force," http://www.ohac.org/merger.html (5/2/99).

Pichon, Victor, 1997, "IRS Health Care Industry Programs and Sanctions," in Kutak Rock, ed., *Sixth Annual Health Care Law Institute*, Omaha, NE: Kutak Rock.

Putnam, Robert, 1993, *Making Democracy Work*, Princeton, NJ: Princeton University Press.

Relman, Arnold S., 1984, "Crisis at General Hospital," *Frontline*, ABC News.

———, "What Market Values Are Doing to Medicine," *The Atlantic Monthly*, March, 99–106.

Relman, Arnold S., and Uwe Reinhardt, 1986, "An Exchange on For-Profit Health Care, in Bradford H. Gray, ed., *For-Profit Enterprise in Health Care*, Washington, DC: National Academy Press.

Social Investment Forum, 1999, http://socialinvest.org/ (11/16/98).

Texas, 1998, V.T.C.A., Health and Safety Code, § 311.045.

The GreenMoney Journal, Spring 1998, "Integrative Investing: How Your Values Make a Difference in the World of Money," http://www.greenmoney.com/gmj/spr98/spr098.htm (12/4/99).

Weissman, Joel, 1996, "Uncompensated Hospital Care: Will It Be There If We Need It?" *Journal of the American Medical Association*, 276(10):823–829.

Wolff, Marie, 1993, "'No Margin, No Mission': Challenge to Institutional Ethics," *Business and Professional Ethics Journal*, 12(2):39.

Wolfson, Jay, and Scott L. Hopes, 1994, "What Makes Tax-Exempt Hospitals Special?" *Healthcare Financial Management*, 48(7):56–60.

Wood, Donna J., 1990, *Business and Society*, New York: HarperCollins Publishers.

Yoder, Sunny G., 1986, "Economic Theories of For-Profit and Not-for-Profit Organizations," in Bradford H. Gray, ed., 1986, *For-Profit Enterprise in Health Care*, Washington, DC: National Academy Press.

Young, Gary, and Kamal R. Desai, 1997, "Does the Sale of Nonprofit Hospitals Threaten Health Care for the Poor?" *Health Affairs*, 16(1):137–141.

3

ADVERTISING AND MARKETING

Between 1992 and 1994 the Woodstock Theological Center convened a seminar of experts to discuss "Ethical Considerations in the Business Aspects of Health Care." One of the major challenges faced by the healthcare system in the United States, they concluded, comes from the influence of market practices:

> The expansion of health care diagnostic and treatment possibilities has also opened up significant profit opportunities to health care professionals and entrepreneurs. Professionals can choose lucrative specialties, or can target niches within their specialties, such as cosmetic plastic surgery or sports medicine, which are especially profitable because many individuals are willing to pay high prices for these services, even if they are specifically excluded from coverage by insurance policies. As a result, the health care field is increasing being influenced by "marketing" practices, and the line between attending to the health care needs of society and selling a consumer product has been increasingly blurred.
>
> (Woodstock, 1995:6)

The members of the Woodstock group were concerned that a commercial model would replace the professional model as the basis of healthcare transactions. According to the professional model, goods and services are not considered subject to commercial transaction because the professional responds to basic human needs with the interest of the client at heart rather than an interest in selling goods or services for a profit. The professional model thus contains an altruistic principle that stands opposed to commercial motives. The transition of health care to a commercial status threatens to undermine the ethical basis of the profession

The commercialization of health care in the United States should come as no surprise, however. Where goods and services can be bought and sold freely and producers can make a profit, market practices will prevail. It's the American way—or at least the dominant trend of American culture at this point. The professional model will now have to find its place within the new commercial world of health care.

In this chapter, some of the more obvious features of the commercialization of health care are addressed. The chapter begins with an analysis of the ethics of advertising in the new commercial context of health care, moves to a discussion of Federal Trade Commission regulations, and concludes with the presentation of a revised marketing perspective for healthcare organizations.

ADVERTISING

One ethical concern raised by the transition of health care to a commercial basis is that purveyors of health services will take advantage of patients by selling them services that are not appropriate to their needs or that they do not need at all. Consider the case of Mrs. L for example. Mrs. L was 87 years old. She was very active and took pride in her appearance and physical fitness. Having seen an advertisement claiming that dental reconstruction could make people appear years younger, she went to the dentist who had placed the ad. He offered her a total dental replacement procedure for $22,000. Mrs. L had had no dental problems at the time; she had lost only two wisdom teeth, and had a couple of root canals and two caps. The treatment was entirely cosmetic. The fact that she was mentally alert and quite capable of choosing how to spend her own money, and of lying about her age (according to her daughter), did not keep her from being a victim of aggressive advertising. Her pride in her appearance had made her vulnerable.

The economic justification of advertising, it is often said, is that it provides information that is necessary for consumers to make intelligent choices. It is ironic that this conventional justification is itself so disingenuous. Who would think of looking to advertising if they really wanted reliable information about products or services? People may look to see what a company is saying about a product or what a product looks like, but if they really want dependable information, they go to articles in reliable publications like *Consumer Reports*.

The basic ethical principles that should govern advertising can be stated in a relatively simple manner. The utilitarian would point out that advertising that is less than honest distorts the market information that is necessary for transactions that will satisfy both providers and consumers. The success of the free market as a means of distributing goods and services is dependent on the free flow of information. This concept is emphasized in health care in the United States, since courts have interpreted agreements reached between healthcare providers and their clients to be subject to informed consent. The adequacy of information is maintained by the requirement that medical providers explain the patient's condition that needs treatment, explain the benefits and risks of the treatment offered, outline the available alternatives (including nontreatment), and assure themselves of the patient's ability to make informed decisions. The problem with advertising is not only that it may create needs that do not exist, as in the case of Mrs. L, but also that it may exaggerate the expected benefits and minimize the risks.

The ethical rationalist would say that deceptive or manipulative advertising violates the integrity of the consumer. The vulnerability of the client must be taken into account. If clients are treated as "ends in themselves," as the Kantian would say, their needs (which may indeed at times include cosmetic needs) ought to be paramount in healthcare transactions, not the desire of providers to sell their services.

The ethical idealist would point out that the commercialization of health care can undermine the trust between providers and their patients that is an integral part of the transaction. The success of the professional relationship, from the idealist perspective, is based on the healthcare provider's trustworthiness. If Mrs. L had discussed this matter further with her own dentist, her fears about her appearance might have been allayed or she might have been offered more reasonable alternatives appropriate to her needs. This presumes, of course, that Mrs. L has a relationship with a dentist and that this dentist is willing and able to take time to discuss her concerns about her appearance and needs. The willingness of dentists and physicians to do this, however, is itself under pressure from the commercialization of health care in which fees are generally charged for procedures completed, not for time spent listening to concerns or giving advice. It is not inconceivable, however, that Mrs. L might have been willing to pay for such a consultation.

When professions that previously rejected advertising begin to allow it, they tend to draw the line at deceptive practices. Consider the following statement from the AMA code of ethics:

> There are no restrictions on advertising by physicians except those that can be specifically justified to protect the public from deceptive practices. A physician may publicize himself or herself as a physician through any commercial publicity or other form of public communication (including any newspaper, magazine, telephone directory, radio, television, direct mail, or other advertising) provided that the communication shall not be misleading because of the omission of necessary

material information, shall not contain any false or misleading statements, and shall not otherwise operate to deceive.

(AMA, 1997:72; see also ADA, 1978)

Prohibiting deception, however, is not the end of the matter: in health care there is also the question of professional responsibility. Traditionally, of course, physicians, lawyers, and members of the clergy are considered professionals rather than vendors. There is still some sense to this distinction, although the concept is losing its power and prestige with the advance of commercialism. A *professional* is a person who can be consulted with reasonable confidence that one can get genuine advice or have access to a certain objective expertise rather than merely being of interest for the potential sale of a product. *Professional responsibility* is the idea that the professional is supposed to have the interests of the client in mind rather than just the sale of services. Arnold Relman, former editor of the *New England Journal of Medicine*, emphasized this point in an article entitled "What Market Values Are Doing to Medicine."

> Although commercial vendors have an obligation to produce a good product and to advertise it without deception, they have no responsibility to consider the consumer's interests—to advise the consumer which product, if any, is really needed, or to worry about those who cannot afford to buy any of the vendors' products.
>
> (Relman, 1992:100)

This is why self-referral and fee splitting are generally considered professionally unethical (AMA, 1997:95–96). Both practices involve conflicts of interest that pit financial interests in the sale of services against the professional duty to give objective opinions and disinterested advice.

Health care is not the only field in which advertising tends to get out of control with respect to larger social goals. Consider the ways in which political advertising and campaign finance practices now threaten to undermine the effectiveness of our political system. The sense of the public interest seems to be all but lost when special interests are allowed to buy access to politicians through campaign contributions. Faced with such threats, society tends to react (unsuccessfully so far with respect to campaign financing) by setting up guidelines. These guidelines can be either voluntary or legally required. In the case of commercial advertising, there are laws against outright deception and specific practices such as *bait and switch*—the practice of luring customers with attractive offers for the purpose of selling them more expensive products.

The mere prohibition of deception, however, can be quite vague. *Deception* is a very broad term that, on the one hand, may be understood to cover only outright lies or, on the other, may be taken to refer to practices that, while not untruthful, may nonetheless influence people who have little or no ability to distinguish fact from fiction. Products and services can be misrepresented artistically, or through the use of technical language (a point noted by the AMA), or simply by guarantees that overstate the probability of satisfaction.

In addition to deception in advertising, which is directed at consumers' knowledge and beliefs, there is the problem of persuasion directed at people's desires. In the late 1950s, two books created something of a popular furor over manipulative advertising. In *The Hidden Persuaders*, Vance Packard claimed that subliminal suggestion by advertising firms was a form of mind control (Packard, 1957). A year later in *The Affluent Society*, John Kenneth Galbraith popularized the notion that the real intent of advertising is not to give information so that people can buy products that satisfy their needs, but to rather create those needs in the first place (Galbraith, 1958). The scare about mind control may be over, but the question must still be asked whether any given advertising attempts to interest potential customers by providing information or whether it also involves an effort to persuade in an affective sense or to create a felt need where none previously existed.

Persuasion, even emotional persuasion, may not be wrong in itself; people sometimes need to be persuaded to do what is in their own interest. But if persuasion is used to create a desire or a felt need for products or services with little or no benefit, it can become manipulative. A number of years ago, my oldest daughter returned from a visit to a dentist with a list of 12 symptoms. If she had any of these symptoms, she had been told, she could probably benefit from new temporomandibular joint (TMJ) corrective procedures. One of her younger sisters, 14 years old at the time, immediately predicted that she would have all 12 by morning. She did!

Creating desires is not the only emotional appeal available to the hidden persuaders. Playing on people's fears is equally important. Writing in *Health Progress* in 1990, Dr. Leonard Weber, director of the Ethics Institute at Mercy College in Detroit, questioned the message communicated by reference to health risks in advertising promoting childbirth services by stressing the medical complications associated with labor and delivery (Weber, 1990). Not quite as threatening but still questionable was a recent TV ad showing a patient with an urgent problem waiting for a long time to be seen by a nurse or physician. The promise was that with the health plan being advertised, this would not happen. Such negative advertising is never appropriate in health care; by nature, it is based on appeals to people's fears that their health or welfare will be endangered if they do not select the services advertised.

DIRECT-TO-CONSUMER DRUG MARKETING

Since 1962 control of the promotion and advertising of prescription drugs has been in the hands of the federal Food and Drug Administration (FDA). The agency established guidelines for listing active and inert ingredients, rules for disclosure of side effects, and the requirement that patients receive full notification with prescriptions. In the 1980s however, pharmaceutical companies began to advertise prescription drugs directly to prospective patients. At first the disclosure rules were strictly applied, but in August 1997, when it had become evident that the broadcast media could not disclose the details usually contained in the fine print of magazine advertisements or product inserts, the FDA issued new guidelines that allowed advertisers to avoid lengthy summaries of potential side effects and contraindications.

The new direct-to-consumer (DTC) advertising has been effective. Writing in the March 1999 issue of the *ACP-ASIM Observer*, Phyllis Maguire reported that the Schering-Plough Corporation spent an estimated $186 million in 1998 to market the antihistamine Claritin to consumers and reaped a $500 million jump in sales from the year before (Maguire, 1999). Direct-to-consumer advertising is also controversial. It has been supported by the American Association of Family Physicians, with a few reservations concerning accuracy, balance, and completeness (AAFP, 1998). The American College of Physicians—American Society of Internal Medicine, on the other hand, says that "direct-to-consumer advertising is not a proper practice . . . that it undermines the patient-physician relationship and often leaves patients confused and misinformed about medications" (ACP-ASIM, 1998). The American Association of Retired Persons is concerned that DTC advertising will add to the rising costs of medications, and other consumer groups have argued that the FDA should require prior clearance (ACP-ASIM, 1998). Finally, the American Association of Hospital Pharmacists says that education about conditions and possible therapies should be permitted, but not information about specific drugs, so it opposes the FDA policy (ACP-ASIM, 1998).

There are certain benefits to DTC advertising. It may encourage conversation between patients and their physicians as patients become better educated about treatments and ask more questions (ACCP, 1995). It may also draw people's attention to their own health status in ways that encourage them to seek treatment. Increased public competition may also lower drug prices. The risks, on the other hand, are that partial information can be misleading and that overly optimistic advertising can actually undermine patients' confidence in their physicians. Indeed, according to Phyllis Maguire, "when doctors try steering patients away from advertised treatments, they find that it's their credibility on the line, not the advertiser's" (Maguire, 1999). There is also the general effect of increasing the amount of medication used in our society.

Case 3.1: Internet Direct-to-Consumer Advertising

Like many other prescription medications, Claritin was originally advertised in public media by name only. Name familiarity or brand recognition is an important element of advertising. In the early 1990s, pharmaceutical companies found that if they advertised only the name of a drug without saying what it was used for, the advertisement was exempt from FDA regulations requiring disclosure of risks and benefits. These so-called reminder ads were confusing to consumers. Schering-Plough, the manufacturer of Claritin, reported getting calls from gynecologists asking why their patients were requesting Claritin (Nordenberg, 1998). Since the FDA revised its rules in 1997, reminder ads along with so-called help-seeking ads telling consumers that help is available for certain conditions and advising them to consult their physician have now largely been supplanted by regular advertisements. Still, within weeks of the publication of the new rules, the FDA ordered an immediate halt to Claritin TV ads because they lacked balance and did not properly direct consumers to full information on the side effects. Specifically, the FDA claimed that the promise that one Claritin tablet can let people "escape the limitations of seasonal allergies" was misleading. Schering-Plough agreed to resolve the matter: the company's current presentation can be found at its Website (Schering-Plough, 1999).

Claritin, however, is offered commercially by retailers that provide much less information. The following information is given on the Medical Center.com Website, a commercial venture of The Pill Box, an online pharmacy in San Antonio, Texas.

Claritin® (Loratadine)—Superior Allergy Relief from Schering-Plough

CLARITIN® provides effective relief from the symptoms of seasonal allergies: itchy, watery eyes; itchy palate; sneezing; and runny nose. CLARITIN® is also effective in relieving the symptoms of itching associated with chronic hives. Unlike all current over-the-counter and some prescription antihistamines (which can make people drowsy), CLARITIN® has no drowsy side effects—so you feel better, not medicated! In studies, the incidence of drowsiness with CLARITIN® was similar to that of placebo (sugar pill) at the recommended dose. Drowsiness may occur if you take more than the recommended dose.

CLICK HERE for an online consultation for a Claritin prescription. Your medical history and patient profile will be reviewed by a Licensed Physician. If approved for a Claritin prescription, we will have your Claritin shipped to you by The Pill Box Pharmacy.

(Medical Center, 1999)

While general ethical principles with regard to advertising can be defined fairly clearly, the jury is out on this particular dispute. The question here is, just how much information should an advertisement be required to present? Presuming that DTC marketing is here to stay, what guidelines might be used to prevent exploitation of vulnerable patients? On the one hand, it might be considered necessary to regulate this form of marketing to protect the doctor–patient relationship from undue external pressure. On the other hand, more consumer information may be better for health care because it may put the consumer in a better position to make informed decisions. Whether the Internet review of the patient's history and prescription by a physician promised in this ad is sufficient is also debatable. Physicians, professional organizations, state medical boards, and the FDA tend to frown on this practice although it is not illegal (Lipsky and Taylor, 1997; Marwick, 1999). Their concern is that the practice undermines the safeguards of the physician–patient relationship and the additional oversight of pharmacy intermediaries. In the past, however, consumer groups argued that many drugs are needlessly controlled, raising prices and adding physician fees.

ETHICAL PERSPECTIVES

Advertising and marketing influence the relationship between healthcare organizations and their customers. Mission statements that mention meeting the health needs of patients acknowledge this important relationship. What must be recognized here, however, is that the relationship is not simply one of a commercial transaction with a vendor of goods and services on the one hand and a consumer on the other. The typical commercial relationship is distorted when it comes to healthcare because of the vast difference in knowledge between the provider and the consumer. Patients do not have sufficient medical knowledge to diagnose their own conditions; they cannot judge their own needs and certainly don't know what medical treatments are appropriate. The consumer is entirely dependent on the provider to give honest and disinterested advice. *Disinterested*, in this context, means that the provider will take the perspective of the patient's interest in obtaining the best health care at the most reasonable cost, and not his or her own interest in selling goods and services. The consumer in this transaction is vulnerable in ways in which consumers in other commercial transactions generally are not.

There is a fiduciary relationship that is implied when the provider–patient relationship is characterized as professional rather than commercial. This relationship is also implied when mission statements of healthcare organizations say that services are "professional" or will be provided "in a professional manner," and it may well be implied in professional accreditation, depending on the standards of the accrediting agencies. The "In Home Health Services Mission Statement" of Newton Memorial Hospital in New Jersey, for example, offers "to provide comprehensive, professional home healthcare to persons in need through highly qualified staff in a progressive, caring environment." It then lists accreditation by the State of New Jersey Health Department, the New Jersey Division of Consumer Affairs, the Community Health Accreditation Program (CHAP), and the Sussex County Chamber of Commerce (Newton, 1996).

This leads to the question of whether healthcare mission statements are more of a form of advertising than statements of commitment to organizational goals. They often present the organization in a way that offers services with the apparent intent of attracting customers. The use of the term *professional* in organizational mission statements is interesting. In common usage, this term distinguishes paid performers, in sports or music for example, from unpaid amateurs. So there is now an element of promotion connected to the term. In health care, although the phrase *professional staff* sometimes refers to everyone except the physician, it retains its basic meaning. It is commonly used to refer to both professional standards and professional review, as in the following statement from the Medical Staff Bylaws of the Department of Veterans Affairs Medical Center in Boston:

The Professional Standards Board acts as the Executive Committee of the Medical Staff for matters concerning appointments, advancements, disciplinary matters and probationary reviews of physicians, dentists, podiatrists, optometrists, nurse anesthetists, physician assistants and expanded function dental auxiliaries.

(VAMC, 1999)

By claiming a professional standing, healthcare organizations and the members of professional associations are implying that they will not take advantage of the vulnerability of their customers in any commercial transaction—that their customers can depend on them to approach the transaction with the interests of the patient as their paramount concern. And this professional perspective applies to advertising and marketing managed by healthcare administrators as well as to the physician's diagnosis or the nurse's care. Advertising and marketing should not take advantage of the consumer's vulnerability.

Although few healthcare organizations do so, it is possible to specify a commitment to fair marketing practices in the context of an organizational goals statement. Advocate Health System does this explicitly:

> *Ethics in marketing.* Guided by our value of Excellence we will protect the confidentiality of our customers and associates who participate in research or other information gathering forums. Guided by our value of Partnership we will exercise responsibility in communications with external and internal audiences and avoid misleading or exaggerated statements. Guided by our value of Equality we will create communications that are responsive and sensitive to our diverse audiences and seek the opinions of our customers and associates in developing our communications.
>
> (Advocate, 1999)

FEDERAL TRADE COMMISSION REGULATIONS

The major source of control and guidance for advertising in the United States is the Federal Trade Commission Act, Section 5, and subsequent policies and guidelines published by the Commission. Regulations govern the substantiation of advertising claims, endorsements, unfairness and deception.

Substantiation requires that advertisers have a "reasonable basis" to support claims or assertions made about products or services. According to one policy statement, of the Federal Trade Commission (FTC),

> when the substantiation claim is express (e.g., "tests prove," "doctors recommend," and "studies show"), the Commission expects the firm to have at least the advertised level of substantiation. Of course, an ad may imply more substantiation than it expressly claims . . . ; in such cases the advertiser must possess the amount and type of substantiation the ad actually communicates to consumers.
>
> (FTC, 1983a)

The FTC maintains that an organization must have substantiation of its claims *before* disseminating advertisements. In its investigative function, the FTC now relies on "nonpublic requests for substantiation directed to individual companies via an informal access letter" rather than engaging in industrywide studies (FTC, 1983a).

The FTC policy on deceptive practices is stated in a 1983 Commission letter to Congressman John Dingell, chairman of the House of Representatives Committee on Energy and Commerce. *Deception* is defined by the FTC as "a misrepresentation, omission or practice that is likely to mislead the consumer acting reasonably in the circumstances, to the consumer's detriment" (FTC, 1983b). The deception only has to be judged "likely" to mislead; proof of actual deception is not necessary. *Detriment* refers to whether deception is likely to change the consumer's conduct or decision.

The standard of whether the "reasonable consumer" might be deceived does not necessarily mean the average person in the general population: "If the representation or practice affects or is directed primarily to a particular group, the Commission examines reasonableness from the perspective of that group" (FTC, 1983b). This can be especially important to healthcare organizations.

> When representations or sales practices are targeted to a specific audience, such as children, the elderly, or the terminally ill, the Commission determines the effect of the practice on a reasonable member of that group. For instance, if a company markets a cure to the terminally ill, the practice will be evaluated from the perspective of how it affects the ordinary member of that group. Thus, terminally ill consumers might be particularly susceptible to exaggerated cure claims. By the same token, a practice or representation directed to a well-educated group, such as a prescription drug advertisement to doctors, would be judged in the light of the knowledge and sophistication of that group.
>
> (FTC, 1983b)

With regard to health matters, we are all somewhat vulnerable. One Commission decision regarding a weight loss product included the following statement:

> It is obvious that dieting is the conventional method of losing weight. But it is equally obvious that many people who need or want to lose weight regard dieting as bitter medicine. To these corpulent consumers the promises of weight loss without dieting are the Siren's call, and advertising that heralds unrestrained consumption while muting the inevitable need for temperance, if not abstinence, simply does not pass muster.
>
> (FTC, 1983a)

As with the substantiation of claims, deception may be either express or implied. And in some cases it may "involve omission of material information, the disclosure of which is necessary to prevent the claim, practice, or sale from being misleading" (FTC, 1983b). In general, the more easily consumers are able to evaluate products and services for themselves, the less the FTC is concerned; but this again implies the need for a greater measure of care on the part of providers of healthcare services.

An *endorsement* is defined by the FTC as a message that reflects the opinions or beliefs of someone other than the advertiser—usually an expert or a well-known person. The FTC guideline for endorsements is that they "must always reflect the honest opinions, findings, beliefs, or experience of the endorser" (FTC, 1980a) and may not state facts that the advertiser cannot substantiate independently or that would be deceptive. An endorser portrayed as a user of a product or service, furthermore, must be and remain an actual user as long as the advertising is disseminated. And people represented as actual customers or consumers must be actual customers or consumers. The same rules apply to the use of research findings in advertising.

In determining what constitutes *unfair practices*, the FTC compares what is being offered with products or services offered by other providers. In a 1980 letter to Congress, the Commission indicated that "unfair methods of competition" include more than practices that substantially injure consumers. Some practices may be "against public policy," and the Commission can appeal to determinations by legislative bodies or the courts for standards by which to judge commercial practices unfair (FTC, 1980b). The Commission is unclear about its practice in this respect, however, and offers only an example of a firm bringing a collection suit in a court that was unreasonably difficult for a defendant to reach. This is not relevant to advertising, but it is an interesting consideration with respect to billing and collections practices. The FTC letter also includes a category of "immoral, unethical, oppressive, or unscrupulous" practices, but it states that the Commission has never relied on this category.

This discussion provides only the general outline of FTC policies and guidelines. Many nuances and details are to be found in Commission cases, some of which are especially relevant to advertising by healthcare organizations. Guidelines often give examples of what *can* be done, as well as what is considered illegal.

A drug company commissions research on its product by a well-known research organization. The drug company pays a substantial share of the expenses of the research project, but the test design is under the control of the research organization. A subsequent advertisement by the drug company mentions the research results as the "findings" of the well-known research organization. The advertiser's payment of expenses to the research organization need not be disclosed in this advertisement. . . . The advertiser's payment will not affect the weight or credibility of the endorsement.

(FTC, 1980b)

REFRACTIVE EYE SURGERY

The FTC has also been active in enforcement. One recent example is its restriction on eye surgery advertising. Refractive eye surgery can improve vision for people who wear glasses or contact lenses by changing the shape of the cornea. The results have been remarkable for many people, and the success rate has been good. This has led to exaggerated claims, however. Advertising copy like "Throw Away Your Glasses" and "The Safe and Easy Alternative" became common when refractive eye surgery was first available. This, in turn, led to unrealistic expectations and disappointment for some people. The FTC eventually concluded that people were not being fully informed in advance about success rates, risks, and long-term benefits since some eye problems could return. The headline message, according to the FTC order, should not be inconsistent with the full disclosure hidden in the fine print. Specifically,

1. Advertising should indicate that patients may need glasses or contact lenses in the future.
2. References to scientific studies should be backed by citations to reputable findings.
3. It should be made clear that excimer laser surgery is, in fact, an invasive procedure.
4. Pain and discomfort cannot be entirely eliminated; advertising should not claim that the procedure is "painless."
5. References to Food and Drug Administration approval of the equipment used are prohibited by law.

(FTC, 1998)

To the credit of the profession, the American Academy of Ophthalmology responded with public information correcting the exaggerated claims (AAO, 1996) and with advice to its members. It is certainly understandable that professionals become enthusiastic about their ability to offer new services that can improve people's lives, but this is exactly when an extra measure of caution about exaggerated claims that may mislead people is necessary. Individual practitioners and provider groups need to examine their own practices. Competitive pressures and exaggerated expectations arise when new procedures become available, and both providers and the public can easily lose perspective.

THE PROS AND CONS OF ADVERTISING

The problems surrounding aggressive advertising in our highly commercial society should not obscure the value of free communication, however. In general, competitive advertising can drive prices down, and it can encourage people to seek care that may be of great benefit to them. From a business perspective, furthermore, the prohibition of advertising in medicine serves the private interests of established providers by making it difficult for new providers to enter the field.

In 1978 the FTC found that provisions of the AMA code restricted competition and that this restriction was a violation of the Federal Trade Commission Act. The FTC therefore required the AMA to drop its ethics code restrictions on advertising of fees, services, or the qualifications of physicians. It also found that the general solicitation of patients should not be prohibited (FTC, 1979). Judicial review by the Federal Circuit Court of Appeals, however, clarified the FTC's order to allow the AMA to restrict false or deceptive advertising and to prohibit uninvited, in-person solicitation of patients "who, because of their particular circumstances, are vulnerable to undue influence" (AMA, 1982:447).

More recently, the FTC took account of this barrier to free trade when it brought an action against the California Dental Association. The Association, according to the FTC, had a code of ethics that limited competition because of its restrictions on advertising and solicitation. The Association's rules prohibited a number of truthful, nondeceptive advertising practices; it had expelled members who violated the rules and had refused membership to others who did not conform. The FTC order required the California Dental Association to change its rules that prohibited ads listing prices and to refrain from interfering with the solicitation of patients (Kutak Rock, 1997).

Studies from the 1980s and 1990s have shown that while consumers generally appreciate hospital advertising, physicians remain skeptical of its benefits and concerned that it will be deceptive or confusing. Bell and Vitaska (1992:7–8) summarized their findings as follows:

> [W]e can conclude that consumers have a generally favorable attitude toward hospital advertising and want information about hospital services, medical programs, and the kinds of doctors available. In contrast, physicians have a generally negative view of hospital advertising and hold substantial reservations about the efficacy of advertising in delivering the information desired by consumers.

This difference may reflect the fact that physicians can retain more control over patients if patient information is limited.

The case against advertising (with reference to HMOs) was presented by Allan S. Brett, MD, in a 1992 article in *The New England Journal of Medicine*. Brett argued that "advertising by HMOs does not expand the options of most potential enrollees, and it may promote the useless movement of patients among health plans." He also cited possible secondary consequences of advertising, "including the creation of unfair expectations among patients, the excessive commercialized portrayal of medical care, and the addition of yet another administrative expense to the health care economy" (Brett, 1992:1356). Psychiatrist Allan Dyer has noted one specific way in which advertising can lead to poorer medical practice. If physicians offering assisted reproduction services advertise their success rates, they may be tempted to recommend implantation of more fertilized ova than would otherwise be medically appropriate. This would lead to a higher success rate, but it would also raise the risk of unwanted multiple pregnancies (Dyer, 1997).

If physicians are quick to point out the risks of advertising, however, they have not been very quick to exercise control over their own practice. In an article in *The Journal of Legal Medicine*, Bradley Olson faults the AMA for including unverified, self-designated specialties along with licensure and board certification information in its own *Directory* (Olson, 1990). In most states physicians can not only designate themselves as specialists, they can also advertise board certification in general fields while representing themselves as specialists in subfields in which they are not certified. Olson notes that Arizona was the first state to place legal controls on physicians representing themselves as specialists in 1989. This does not speak well for a profession that otherwise insists on self-regulation. In fact, self-regulation, as suggested by Allan Brett in the article cited above, could run the risk of antitrust complications to which state regulations would be immune (Olson, 1990).

Case 3.2: The Paradox of Success

Effective advertising can also lead to ethical issues of market selectivity. Consider the following example. A not-for-profit managed care plan attempted to respond to the needs of its members. Its advertising strategy was to present itself as the health care plan that does everything it can to serve its members. The strategy included a strong emphasis on its nonprofit status and its inclusion of elected members on its governing board and treatment review committee. The organization of this plan under state mutual insurance regulations provides that plan profits will be distributed to members as dividends. As new drugs and combinations of drugs became available for AIDS patients, the plan made them available even though they were classified as experimental. While full and aggressive treatment for AIDS patients was not emphasized in plan advertising, its availability soon became known in the gay and lesbian community. Unintentionally, the advertising campaign came to have special meaning in this community, and enrollments from this market sector increased.

While the increase in memberships demonstrated that the marketing strategy was effective, it also presented certain problems. The larger gay and lesbian percentage of plan members might affect the financial stability of the plan through higher costs for treating this population. The fiscal impact could be positive, however. Although the data were not fully reliable, the gay and lesbian sector of the population was believed to have a higher median household income than the general population. In a market where costs were rising, gay and lesbian people would be valued customers who might be willing to pay higher membership fees. The question of the financial impact of enrolling a higher percentage of gay and lesbian members is an actuarial question. Ethically, however, one can ask whether this information ought to be considered at all. Should healthcare advertising either attract or avoid any sector of the public on the grounds of sexual orientation? One can imagine the public offense if minorities or certain religious groups were considered in this way. This is an instance of a general problem that faces healthcare insurance plans and has an impact on advertising decisions: if the plan serves the specific needs of people with particular health conditions effectively, its own success may lead to an influx of enrollees with a higher level of plan use, and this, in turn, may raise the cost for others.

THE IMPORTANCE OF MARKETING FROM AN ETHICAL PERSPECTIVE

Advertising has acquired its less than flattering reputation largely because it has become separated from many of the other aspects of marketing; and marketing itself has often been understood only in terms of advertising. Marketing strategy is a much larger concept—one that, rightly understood, can be an important focus of creative ethical consideration and an essential part of the mission of a healthcare organization.

Marketing, as it is now conceived by business strategists, refers to a relationship between providers and customers that is much wider than just convincing customers to purchase goods as offered. It addresses the needs of the customers and the design of the product. A helpful approach to this wider notion of marketing is to consider one of its better-known aspects: market research. Market research may be done to determine the advertising strategy, that is, to gain a better understanding of prospective customers in order to persuade them to purchase the product. But market research may also be undertaken for product design and development—to determine the needs of potential customers in order to create a product or service that will effectively meet those needs. Understood in this way, the purpose of market research in health care is to assist in redesigning the product—the healthcare delivery system—to allow it to do its job better. The market analyst would thus be concerned with such problems as how long patients have to wait in emergency rooms, the communication skills of physicians and nurses, and ultimately whether the customer—the patient—is given the opportunity to be fully informed and participate in decisions regarding his or her treatment and care. The analyst should also be concerned about how families are approached regarding organ donation and about how effective discharge planning is from the patient's perspective. Good marketing can be good clinical ethics.

In a recent textbook on marketing, for example, Nickels and Wood (1997) point out the way in which the definition of marketing has changed over the last few decades. In 1948 the American Marketing Association defined marketing as "the performance of business activities directed toward, and incident to, the flow of goods from producer to consumer" (4). By 1985, however, the field was understood in a way that was much more integral to the organization. According to this new understanding, marketing is "the process of planning and executing the conception, pricing, promotion and distribution of ideas, goods and services to create exchanges that satisfy individual and organizational objectives" (4). Nickels and Wood go on to explain their own advocacy of marketing as "the process of establishing and maintaining mutually beneficial long-term relationships among organizations and their customers, employees and other stakeholders" (4–5). As the relationship with all stakeholders has replaced the customer focus in marketing, two-way communication has replaced promotion, and in the process, ethical aspects have become central. This has allowed marketing to direct its attention not only to the promotion of products but also to the determination of people's needs for which goods and services must be developed (McKenna, 1991; Morgan and Hunt, 1994). My point here is that the closer healthcare market analysts come to researching the actual needs of patients, the closer they come to some of the crucial issues of clinical and organizational ethics.

Market strategists now need to focus as much on the design of the product as on the needs of the customer. It is as much the task of the marketing division of a healthcare organization to tell the organization what the customer wants as it is to convince the customer to purchase what the organization has to sell. In fact, the marketing specialist should be a key contributor to operations management, strategic planning, and institutional development. The perspective of the marketing specialist in many respects should be the managerial perspective that has the closest link to the customer and thereby to the community. The market analyst has the specific task of representing (re-presenting to management) the interests of some of the healthcare organization's most important stakeholders. Good marketing can also be good organizational ethics. If the mission of an organization is to address the healthcare needs of a community (and this is quite often the first principle of an institutional mission statement), then it would seem reasonable that a marketing division should be responsible for assessing and evaluating those needs.

Marketing, as distinct from advertising, is thus on the track of a new philosophy. It begins with finding out what the customer needs, moves to planning and developing products and services that will satisfy those needs, and only then to promotion and distribution. From the perspective of this philosophy, all organizational planning and operations should be customer-oriented and all marketing activities should be organizationally coordinated. Thus, it is essential to have marketing managers involved in healthcare organizational ethics programs, both because they may benefit from the ethical perspectives the program can provide, and because they are likely to have insights into specific ethical issues.

CONCLUSIONS

Health care has emerged from a culture of professional service in which advertising was deemed inappropriate marketplace competition. Special care is needed to keep vulnerable individuals—people at a disadvantage because of serious health conditions—from being victimized by aggressive market tactics. The professional perspective that once defended patients from undue manipulation is now under heavy pressure from commercialization. Federal guidelines are developing, but healthcare organizations must also make it clear in their policies and practices that advertising should present helpful information and not take advantage of human frailties. Efficient marketing programs begin with research on people's actual needs and then foster the development of products or services to meet those needs.

REFERENCES

AAFP (American Academy of Family Physicians), 1998, "Compendium of AFFP Positions on Selected Health Issues: Advertising," http://www.aafp.org/policy/3.html (3/20/99).

AAO (American Academy of Ophthalmology), 1996, "Refractive Eye Surgery," http://www.eyenet.org/public/ref_surg/ref_surg.html (3/7/98)

ACCP (American College of Clinical Pharmacy), 1995, "Direct-to-Consumer Promotion" [letter], FDA; Docket No. 95N-0227, Washington, DC: Food and Drug Administration.

ACP-ASIM (American College of Physicians–American Society of Internal Medicine), 1998, "Policy: Direct to Consumer Advertising for Prescription Drugs," http://www.acponline.org/hpp/pospaper/dtcads.htm (12/4/99).

ADA (American Dental Association), 1978, "Principles of Ethics," http://csep.iit.edu/codes/ada-d.htm (2/24/98)

Advocate (Advocate Health Care), 1999, "Advocate Health Care Ethics Statement," Oak Brook, Illinois, http://www.advocatehealth.com/about/faith/healing/chuw8.html (4/29/99).

AMA (*American Medical Association v. Federal Trade Commission*), 1982, 638 F2d 443–457.

AMA (American Medical Association), 1997, *Code of Medical Ethics: Current Opinions and Annotations*, 1996–1997 edition, Chicago: American Medical Association.

Bell, Jack A., and Charles R. Vitaska, 1992, "Who Likes Hospital Advertising—Consumer or Physician?" *Journal of Health Care Marketing*, 12(2):2–8.

Brett, Allan S., 1992, "The Case Against Persuasive Advertising by Health Maintenance Organizations," *New England Journal of Medicine*, 326(20):1353–1357.

Dyer, Allan R., 1997, "Ethics, Advertising, and Assisted Reproduction: The Goals and Methods of Advertising," *Women's Health Issues*, 7(3):143–148.

FTC (Federal Trade Commission), 1979, 94 F.T.C. 701.

———, 1980a, "FTC Guides Concerning Use of Endorsements and Testimonials in Advertising," http://www.ftc.gov/bcp/guides/endorse.htm (3/11/98).

——, 1980b, "FTC Policy Statement on Unfairness," http://www.ftc.gov/bcp/guides/ad1unfar.htm (3/11/98).

——, 1983a, "FTC Policy Statement Regarding Advertising Substantiation," http://www.ftc.gov/bcp/guides/ad3subst.htm (3/11/98).

——, 1983b, "Policy Statement on Deception," http://www.ftc.gov/bcp/guides/ad2decpt.htm (3/11/98).

——, 1998, "In the Matter of Summit Technology, Inc., a Corporation, and VISX, Inc., a Corporation, DOCKET NO. 9286, AGREEMENT CONTAINING CONSENT ORDER TO CEASE AND DESIST," http://www.ftc.gov/os/1998/9808/d09286viagr.htm (8/21/98).

Galbraith, John Kenneth, 1958, *The Affluent Society*, New York: Houghton Mifflin.

In re AMA (American Medical Association), 1982, 94 *F.T.C.* 701 (1979), aff'd, 638 F.2d, 443, affirmed 445 U.S. 676, rehearing denied, 456 U.S. 966.

Kutak Rock [law firm], 1997, *Sixth Annual Health Law Institute*, Omaha, NE: Kutak Rock.

Lipsky, Martin S., and Christine A Taylor, 1997, "The Opinions and Experiences of Family Physicians Regarding Direct-to-Consumer Advertising," *Journal of Family Practice*, 45(6):495–499.

Maguire, Phyllis, 1999, "How Direct-to Consumer Advertising Is Putting the Squeeze on Physicians," *ACP-ASIM Observer* (American College of Physicians—American Society of Internal Medicine), March, 1999 http://www.acponline.org/journals/news/mar99/squeeze.htm (12/9/99).

Marwick, Charles, 1999, "Several Groups Attempting Regulation of Internet Rx," *Journal of the American Medical Association*, 281:975–976.

McKenna, Regis, 1991, *Relationship Marketing*, Reading, MA: Addison-Wesley.

Medical Center, 1999, "Medical Center.com," The Pill Box Pharmacy, San Antonio, TX, http://www.medicalcenter.net/claritin.htm (3/20/99).

Morgan, Robert M., and Shelby D. Hunt, 1994, "The Commitment-Trust Theory of Relationship Marketing," *Journal of Marketing*, 58(3):20–38.

Newton (Newton Memorial Hospital), 1996, "Mission Statement," Newton, NJ, http://www.itsyourlife.com/inhomeh.htm (1/20/99).

Nickels, William G., and Marian Burk Wood, 1997, *Marketing: Relationships, Quality, Value*, New York: Worth Publishers.

Nordenberg, Tamar, 1998, "Direct to You: TV Drug Advertisements That Make Sense," FDA Consumer, http://www.fda.gov/fdac/features/1998/198_ads.html (12/4/98).

Olson, Bradley J., 1990, "Physician Specialty Advertising: The Tendency to Deceive?" *The Journal of Legal Medicine*, 11:351–371.

Packard, Vance, 1957, *The Hidden Persuaders*, New York: David McKay.

Relman, Arnold S., 1992, "What Market Values Are Doing to Medicine," *The Atlantic Monthly*, March, 99–106.

Schering-Plough, 1999, "Claritin," Kenilworth, NJ, http://www.claritin.com/index.php3 (5/3/99).

VAMC (Veterans Affairs Medical Center), 1999, "Medical Staff Bylaws and Rules," Boston, http://www.visn1.org/boston/bylaws.htm (12/4/99).

Weber, Leonard J., 1990, "The Business of Ethics," *Health Progress*, 71:87–88, 102.

Woodstock (Woodstock Theological Center), 1995, *Ethical Considerations in the Business Aspects of Health Care*, Washington, DC: Georgetown University Press.

4

MANAGED CARE

Conflict of interest is a key concept in business ethics (Margolis, 1979) and in healthcare organizational ethics (JCAHO, 1998:77–83). A conflict of interest exists whenever a decision maker has a motive for making a decision that is not in the interest of the organization of which he or she is an agent (an organizational conflict of interest) or of a client or patient (a professional conflict of interest). The most common conflicts of interest are those between organizational or professional obligations and the personal interests of the decision maker—for example, when a physician refers a patient to a home health agency in which he has a financial interest. But a conflict can also occur between a professional's obligation to a client and his or her other obligations: a physician may need to spend extra time explaining a procedure to a patient, while the organization expects her to be seeing other patients.

The concept of a conflict of interest is used in this chapter as a means of addressing the major ethical problems surrounding managed care. Conflict of interest is key to managed care issues because the advent of managed care has brought with it a new system of incentives. This is only one way of approaching the ethical dimension of this transition, but since managed care has created new conflicts of interest in medicine, it is central to an understanding of the some of the most crucial ethical issues (Arras and Steinbock, 1999).

MANAGED CARE

Managed care is a form of health insurance in which the delivery of care to a patient is under the control of a physician (or allied professional) case manager. Typically the physician provides the patient's primary care and oversees referrals to specialists or other providers for additional care. The care that is offered to a participant in a managed care plan is only what is deemed appropriate by the managing physician and approved by the plan. As a healthcare delivery system, managed care also concerns efficiency, coordination of care, preventive care, early detection, wellness programs, and many other possible benefits for members. But at this point in the evolution of the U.S. healthcare system, the financial aspects are central: managed care is about money.

Under the indemnity insurance system, physicians' charges and hospital bills were paid by the insurer. Physicians could charge their customary fees, and hospitals were supposed to be reimbursed for their costs. There were no incentives to control costs. The patient would request that "everything possible" be done, and the physician, who had no incentives to do otherwise, would usually comply. The problem with the economics of this system was that neither the consumer nor the provider had any reason to be concerned with the cost because someone else, the insurer, was paying the bill.

In the 1970s, when healthcare costs were on a sharp inflationary trend (as high as 20% annually in the hospital sector) and health insurance bills to employers were doubling every five years, health maintenance organizations (HMOs) became an attractive option. The HMO idea was that if a company paid a set annual fee to a provider group to cover the health care of its employees, the providers would have an economic incentive to control costs and the physicians and hospitals involved in the plan would be able to make a profit by keeping the cost down. The theory was that with a prepaid health plan there would no longer be any incentive to overtreat patients, and there would be an added incentive to offer preventive care and screening for early detection of health problems. And to a large extent, the new system worked (Hillman et al., 1989).

Managed care developed out of the HMO movement when insurance plans in the 1980s adopted the case management procedures of HMOs. In terms of controlling costs, this strategy also worked. According to the Centers for Disease Control, "for employers with fewer than 500 employees, health-care costs declined in 1994 for the first time in a decade; this decrease resulted almost entirely from a shift of health insurance from traditional fee-for-service indemnity plans to less costly managed care plans" (CDC, 1995:4). Under this new system, the economic incentives were, in fact, reversed. Rather than getting paid according to how much care could be given (or how sick the patient was), providers would now be rewarded for controlling costs.

Once the cat of economic incentives was out of the bag, however, healthcare finance schemes exploded in all directions. Employers found that they could contract directly with provider groups and save administrative expenses by by-passing the insurance companies; insurance companies and managed care plans found that they could contract with physicians and hospitals (preferred pro-viders) for a set schedule of fees; insurance companies could require second opinions or preauthorization for expensive treatment; and, most important, man-aged care organizations (MCOs) could be run on a for-profit basis by indepen-dent corporations (as well as by physician groups, hospital groups, nonprofit organizations, and insurance companies). As a result, there are now so many different types of healthcare financing systems that it is difficult to categorize them in any simple scheme. But they are all variations on a theme: physicians and hospitals get paid set fees, and patients have to have services approved. The term *managed care* originally referred to the fact that the members of the plan would have their health care managed; but the new financial mechanisms actu-ally manage the providers just as much as the patients. The change from the fee-for-service indemnity insurance system to the many varieties of managed care constitutes a major revolution in health care (Zoloth-Dorfman and Rubin, 1995).

The ethical issues involved in managed care are directly related to the eco-nomic incentives in the new system. Under managed care, the provider has a duty not only to the patient but also to the plan itself—a duty to control costs. For physicians, this creates a conflict of interest in which their obligation to the plan (to implement cost controls) may conflict with their obligation to their patients (Lemieux-Charles et al., 1993). This conflict is evident in the most common complaint about managed care: that plan approval for treatment is withheld contrary to medical advice. Consider the following story from a Cali-fornia surgeon, as reported by Laurie Zoller-Dorfman and Susan Rubin:

I had made a routine call to my patient's HMO to get approval for surgical removal of what I thought were pilar tumors on the patient's scalp. The HMO physician consultant, a long-retired physician (not a dermatologist), approved the surgery, but then asked me what I intended to do with the tissue once I had removed it. Startled, I told him that I intended to send it to the lab for pathology to examine, as always. He advised me that the HMO would not approve payment for pathology, since the tumors were benign. I informed him that there was a remote chance of malignancy, as reported in the literature, though the odds were thin. With this in mind, it was my opinion as a board certified dermatologist, a board certified dermatopathologist, and a caring physician, that an inexpensive histopathological confirmation that the tumors were benign was not an unreasonable request and was clearly the standard of care in the community. Notwithstanding, the request was denied. When asked what he suggested I do with the tumors, the HMO consultant replied that I could do whatever I wished, submit them or trash them, but payment would not be forthcom-ing. I informed my patient that the HMO had refused to pay for the pathology exam, but I felt so strongly that the exam was indicated that I would send the specimen to the lab at my own expense. And, on the advice of my liability carrier, I followed up by documenting my communication with the HMO and sending copies to my local medical society. . . .

(Zoller-Dorfman and Rubin, 1995:342)

The surgeon then explained the financial arrangements of the HMO and the consequences of his actions as follows:

All of the physicians on the HMO panel have 10 percent of their reimbursement withheld routinely until the end of the year when they are rated against their peers regarding practice patterns (utilization, prescription of non-generic drugs, et cetera) and rewarded or penalized accordingly. The maximum reward a physician can receive back is 150 percent of his initial "10 percent withheld"; the maximum penalty is a 65 percent loss of the 10 percent withheld. I received my first-ever negative rating on quality based on this incident, and I was given the maximum financial penalty. In a letter from the HMO I was told, "The forwarding of a copy of your letter to the patient and to [the local medical society] suggests strongly that you are not acting in a collegial mode with us in this matter. [We] sincerely [wish] to partner with [our] providers in the deliverance of quality necessary care. In order to do this there must be a mutual trust and understanding of our respective roles. Medical necessity is determined on the basis of sound science. Your communication regarding this matter will become part of our Quality Management file." I am now concerned about being removed from the HMO panel, which provides me with a large proportion of my referrals.

(Zoller-Dorfman and Rubin, 1995:342–343)

The consequences of this new healthcare delivery and finance system have been widely reported (Gorman, 1998). Since the early 1990s, stories of patients being denied needed care or having to wait so long for approval that their conditions deteriorated have been common. MCOs have been struggling to serve their customers' needs while still keeping costs under control, but the battle is not over yet.

To say that managed care introduces a conflict of interest where no conflict previously existed is not entirely correct (Rodwin, 1993). Physicians did indeed have conflicts of interest under the fee-for-service system. The conflicts, however, were of the sort that led to overtreatment because physicians got paid more for overtreating than for undertreating. So it seemed that the conflict was harmless to the patient—unless, as was evident at times, unnecessary surgery or treatment was harmful. Harmless or not, the conflict was there: it was just ignored. Although the rather ineffective requirement of second opinions was designed to overcome this conflict of interest, physicians were not in the habit of recusing themselves from performing procedures on the grounds that they stood to profit from their own diagnoses. The conflicts of interest in the fee-for-service system and the consequent inflation of healthcare costs did in fact lead to demands for reform in terms of case review, to tissue monitoring, and eventually to the DRG system. The conflicts did not, however, put the patient's health at risk, so they were ignored by the public until the cost of health care itself became an issue.

The reversal of economic incentives under managed care, however, has reversed the situation with regard to conflicts of interest. Since the physician now has a responsibility to the MCO to contain costs, and may furthermore have his or her income tied to performance with regard to cost containment, the incentive is to undertreat rather than overtreat. And the patient is at risk of receiving too little rather than too much health care. Note that the patient has no more power than under the previous system, that is, the patient is no more capable of determining independently what health care he or she needs than before. Here, however, the patient is more at risk because the economic interests involved are in favor of curtailing care rather than overtreatment.

While MCOs presumably do not intend to deny patients needed care, the conflict of interests under MCO plans is intentional; the control mechanisms are explicit. Physicians are paid per patient rather than per visit, so if they see the same patient too often, they earn less. Part of their compensation may be withheld until a practice review shows that they have met cost containment objectives. They may receive bonuses at certain times calculated directly on the basis of their performance in containing costs. Or after a performance review, they may be dropped from the plan if they have a contractual relationship, or terminated, if they are employed by the plan.

A second type of control measure is practice guidelines. As in the case of the California surgeon, reported above, MCO plans generally establish clinical guidelines and require plan approval for certain treatments. This may take a clinical decision out of the hands of the physician, but it does not remove the conflict of interests. In fact, it intensifies the conflict because the physician is prevented from ordering what is in the best interests of the patient. How strong these incentives are and how dangerous the conflict of interest is to the patient vary with the plan.

REMEDIES

The ethical problems that arise from managed care are serious. They include the direct withholding of care from patients, the compromising of providers' professional responsibility (nurses as well as physicians) to act in their patients' best interests, and even the overriding of physicians' clinical judgments. Yet the cost containment that managed care can achieve is essential. The American healthcare system has been out of control financially for years, absorbing an inordinately large percentage of the gross domestic product in the United States compared with other highly industrialized nations while producing no better results (Cockerham, 1997). The question, therefore, is whether cost containment can be attained under ethically acceptable conditions. To answer this question, we must look at what can be done to control, eliminate, or render harmless the conflicts of interest that make the system ethically unacceptable. A number of proposals have been made.

Medical Professionalism

The ethical significance of those occupations that are customarily considered professions is that their practitioners are committed to advancing the interests of their clients without regard to their own interests. According to the AMA code of ethics:

> The duty of patient advocacy is a fundamental element of the physician–patient relationship that should not be altered by the system of health care delivery in which physicians practice. Physicians must continue to place the interests of their patients first. When managed care plans place restrictions on the care that physicians in the plan may provide to their patients . . . physicians must advocate for any care they believe will materially benefit their patients.
>
> (AMA, 1997:126)

If this professional ethic can be enhanced and reinforced through education and strong professional associations, it has been suggested, physicians will be able to withstand the pressures of managed care plans to cut costs at the expense of their patients' health (Christensen, 1996; Emmanuel and Brett, 1993; IHA, 1998; Woodstock, 1995).

Reliance on the professional commitment of individual physicians to overcome the economic pressure exerted by MCOs may be somewhat naive, however. The guidelines and incentives of MCOs, as illustrated by the case of the California surgeon, can threaten not only one's income but also one's position. The surgeon in this case took action to defend his professional judgment and to fulfill his obligation to his patient. But given the consequences, will physicians in such situations be likely to continue to hold the line? Physicians themselves seem to be worried by this power struggle. The AMA recently approved the development of a labor union for managed care and other institution-based physicians with the express purpose of strengthening physicians' advocacy. Medical professionalism is up against a very powerful opponent: I wouldn't bet on Hippocrates.

Full Disclosure

A common way of reducing the harmful effects of conflicts of interest is to have a rule requiring full disclosure of people's interests. This is common in governmental operations. I was once vice president of a health systems agency that regularly discussed applications for state certificates of need. Many members of the committee were healthcare providers, and on occasion the agency had to deal with a matter that directly affected some of their business interests. It was expected that members would disclose this conflict of interests and would not vote on the issue before the committee. A similar disclosure procedure would help to clarify the situation under managed care. Patients should know about the financial arrangements their physicians have with managed care plans and about any guidelines that control the physician's practice (AMA, 1997:126–127). Ideally, people enrolling in a plan should know in advance just what the plan does or does not cover. Prospective members would then have the choice of accepting the conditions or finding another plan. Competition between plans would then presumably weed out providers that curtail treatment to the detriment of patients.

While such full disclosure may seem effective in theory, however, it is not always sufficient in practice. Lay people have little experience with which to judge whether their physicians' contractual arrangements are likely to compromise their clinical judgment. They have even less ability to judge whether specific practice guidelines are appropriate or whether the rules would deny them care they might need. The AMA's supposition that under full disclosure "patients may then determine whether an appeal is appropriate, or whether they wish to seek care outside the plan for treatment alternatives that are not covered" (AMA, 1997:127), is inadequate. This may be effective for upper-middle-class, well-educated patients, but it is entirely unrealistic for most people. Employers may only offer a choice among inconsequential alternatives, and most people cannot afford out-of-plan care. Full disclosure in the absence of any power to change the options has little effect (Rodwin, 1993:213–219).

Informed Consent

The AMA (1997) and other professional organizations have strongly asserted that the provision of health care under managed care systems should not interfere with informed consent or other patient rights. The Midwest Bioethics Center, for example, has drawn up a list of the rights that ought to be assured to members of managed care plans. The list includes the basic elements of informed consent; specifically, patients should be assured the right "to have any proposed procedure or treatment explained in language(s) the member can understand, including descriptions of: the nature and purpose of the treatment, possible benefits, known side effects, risks or draw-backs, the recovery process, including potential problems associated with recovery, likelihood of success, optional procedures or treatments, including non-treatment, and any additional costs for which the patient may be responsible" (Biblo et al., 1996:MC13). The point is well taken; informed consent has been a mainstay of patients' rights in bioethics since the field began. And it is legally required in most jurisdictions, so this safeguard has the backing of the state and powerful enforcement mechanisms. In fact, close attention to this principle could help to minimize the risks associated with the managed care conflict of interest if patients were fully informed about possible treatments that the plan does not cover, as well as those it does.

While informed consent is one of the strongest safeguards against the limitation of treatment under managed care, it is not likely to solve the problem in a definitive way. It requires strong consumer advocacy in terms of knowing how to judge among alternative courses of treatment. The nature of health care, however, is such that patients are unable to make these judgments without professional help. It is too easy for providers to convince patients that they should choose the care that is recommended by the plan. Managed care plans, furthermore, may find that they can inform patients about better (and more expensive) treatments without offering to cover them because competitive plans don't cover them either.

Scientific Practice Guidelines

One way to answer the question of who is getting adequate treatment is to have better information on outcomes. If the actual success rate of dialysis for patients with acute renal failure were more widely known, for example, this treatment would probably not be offered as often as it is, and patients would be spared the pain and suffering associated with this often futile procedure (MacKay and Moss, 1997). It would then be reasonable for an MCO to have a practice guideline stating that dialysis will not be offered to patients for whom it holds little or no hope of benefit. As scientific outcome data become available for a wider range of medical procedures, practice guidelines based on these data should reduce dispute about which treatments are beneficial.

While better outcome data will help to minimize disputes, however, medicine will never be entirely a science. The data, furthermore, always come in probabilistic form—such and such a chance of success under such and such conditions. Whether this chance of success is sufficient to warrant a given procedure will still be a matter of judgment, and opinions of physicians often differ from published practice guidelines (Chin, 1997).

Appeals Procedures

Closely associated with the establishment of clinical guidelines is the question of patients appealing denial of care. There can be little objection to the idea that any managed care plan ought to have a procedure for members to file grievances and appeals (Biblo et al., 1996). The devil here is in the details. Who will hear the grievance: plan administrators, physicians employed by the plan, a panel of practitioners, or a committee including plan members? It has been suggested that for an appeals board to have any real power and credibility, it must be composed of people external to the plan. Another suggestion is that the state should establish a public appeals board that would have the power to mandate that a plan pay for treatment it judges appropriate. Government involvement is not always the most efficient mechanism, but it is certainly an alternative. Recognizing the value of separating medical decision making from financial considerations, the AMA has insisted that practicing physicians must be included in any MCO panel that sets clinical guidelines (AMA, 1995). In fact, the AMA went further, proposing legislation in 1994 that would require MCOs to establish separate medical staff structures similar to those of hospitals (AMA, 1994). With any appeals procedure, of course, one has to have the knowledge, the ability, and the time to go through the process. The prospect of members hiring lawyers to bring their cases before an official appeals board, whether within the plan or externally, is not a happy one. Recent legal cases have involved claims that patients died or were irreparably harmed while awaiting appeals within managed care plans.

Controlling Financial Incentives

The conflict of interest inherent in managed care could also be reduced by restricting the financial incentives involved. The risk of income loss to a physician based on his or her clinical practice compared with plan expectations can range from small to large, and the conflict of interest will vary accordingly. The federal government has taken a stand on this issue. In 1992 the Health Care Financing Administration issued rules for the Medicare and Medicaid programs limiting the percentage of a physician's compensation that could be tied to performance criteria (*Federal Register,* 1992;57:59024–59040). This solution may help, but it addresses only one aspect of the conflict of interest situation and will thus have limited effect.

Patients' Bill of Rights

The fear that cost cutting will reduce the availability or quality of health care has led to calls for government control. The first legislation to be passed in some states was a response to the so-called drive-through delivery limits of some managed care plans under which a woman giving birth was entitled to only one night in the hospital. Some state legislatures required any MCO plan offering health care in the state to provide a longer hospital stay. This legislation was something of a warning: it would clearly be impractical to write detailed practice guidelines into law, but the public had shown that it could and would respond to what it saw as plan limits that endangered people's health with specific requirements.

Many of the controls mentioned here were included in the various patients' rights bills presented to Congress in 1998 and 1999. Proposals included the following provisions (S. 1890, 1998):

a. Emergency care is to be covered without authorization and regardless of provider when a prudent lay-person would believe that his or her health is in immediate danger,

b. Members are to be allowed a choice of providers from among those in the plan that are available,

c. Women may choose an Obstetrician/Gynecologist as primary care physician or must have access to an Obstetrician/Gynecologist without pre-authorization,

d. Members are to be referred to specialists appropriately,

e. Continuity of care and transition for treatment plans is assured if the managed care coverage is terminated,

f. Treatment under clinical trials must be covered,

g. Prescriptions not listed in the plan formulary must be covered if medically necessary,

h. Plans must provide an adequate number and variety of specialists,

i. Plans cannot discriminate on the basis of race, sex, ethnicity, sexual orientation, genetic information, etc.,

j. Every plan must maintain a quality assurance program including drug utilization and must publish quality data in a standardized form,

k. Managed care plans are subject to full disclosure regarding benefits, access, out-of-area and emergency coverage, authorization and grievance procedures, utilization review and provider compensation,

l. Plans must also have a grievance process and a procedure for hearing appeals on denials of care with the possibility of appeal to an external arbitrator,

m. Gag rules are prohibited,

n. Providers contracting with managed care organizations may not be subjected to retaliation for disclosing information about the plan and its operations, or for participating in any legal procedure or investigation,

o. Plans that cover breast surgery for cancer must also cover reconstructive surgery.

The list is long, but legislators apparently feel that it must cover the most common abuses that are generated under the new managed care incentives. Long as it is, the patients' bill of rights is directed to preventing abuse rather than to removing conflicts of interest. While such federal regulation may not be the best way to assure quality health care, and will surely entangle the healthcare system further in bureaucratic paperwork, it must be realized that consumers have no other options. Regulations that set standards, furthermore, will help to create a more level playing field in this competitive market between plans that want to operate under high ethical standards and those that ignore patients' rights for the sake of increasing the profit margin.

Whether any of these measures, or any combination of them, will sufficiently reduce the conflicts of interest inherent in the managed care system or minimize their effects remains to be seen. The law can establish minimal ethical standards, but managed care policies and practices will have to be judged ethically beyond mere compliance with law. The extent to which business and governmental entities that pay for health benefits can rein in these excesses of managed care is another avenue that has not been fully explored (Anderson, 1997).

Evaluating ethical guidelines for managed care is no easy matter. My impression so far is that voluntary actions and good will, such as most of the steps proposed by the Midwest Bioethics Center project (Biblo et al., 1996), will not be forceful enough in the long run. Among the "Rights and Responsibilities" proposed by this project are a number of points that are already covered under current laws in most states. These include provisions against discrimination, access to medical records, informed consent guidelines, surrogate decision maker provisions, advance directive powers, and confidentiality of medical records. These rights certainly need to be protected in managed care settings, but they are largely required by law already and will not eliminate the conflicts of interest inherent in the structure.

Other points suggested by the Midwest Bioethics Center are well taken, but too vague or too much dependent on good will to be enforced: treating members with respect, minimizing pressures to make treatment decisions on economic grounds, and responding to reasonable requests from members fall into this category. Other ethical requirements noted by the Midwest Bioethics Center project are right on target: the opportunity to choose providers from an adequate panel, the opportunity to appeal decisions, and full disclosure of plan guidelines. The problem here, as with managed care in general, is one of mandating the proposed practices forcefully enough to withstand the financial pressures that come from the competitive economics of health care or the expectations of stockholders for a high return on investment. Structural problems require structural remedies. Organizational ethicists ought to be skeptical of reliance on voluntary efforts. A similar effort, the "Code of Ethics for Managed Care in Colorado" produced by the Rocky Mountain Center for Healthcare Ethics, also addresses discrimination, disclosure, confidentiality, professional obligations, and membership involvement in decision making (RMCHE, 1997). Like the Midwest Bioethics Center project, however, this is also a voluntary approach.

The issue of conflict of interest in managed care has a double focus. It certainly involves the risk to plan members that the health care available to them will be inappropriately limited because of the plan's cost containment measure. The other side of the coin, and just as important to the ethics of managed care, is the nature of the contract between the plan and its professional providers. It is, in fact, the same conflict of interests that is crucial here. Professional contracts, therefore, need to be considered from the perspective of putting physicians, nurses, and other professional providers in a situation in which they bear the burden of the conflict. The much publicized gag rule is a good example. It is offensive because it is really the MCO plan that limits the treatment alternatives; but by preventing physicians from discussing treatment alternatives not offered under the plan, the professional contract forces physicians to bear the burden of the conflict of interest by being dishonest with their patients. The plan, in effect, wants members to believe that it is the physicians' professional judgment that is limiting their care to certain alternatives rather than the practice guidelines of the plan itself. So professional contracts need to be reviewed with respect to the ethical consequences of the conflicts of interest inherent in managed care as well.

THE EVOLUTION OF A HEALTHCARE SYSTEM

Managed care is now the focus of the U.S. healthcare system itself. We are in the midst of a major social change, the outcome of which is not yet clear. It is in fact more of a revolution than an evolution because control has shifted from professional providers of health care to institutional administrators. The central issue in this transition is the question of whether cost containment can be achieved without diminishing the quality of care. The issue has an important ethical dimension: what limitations on care will people find morally acceptable? The locus of this issue, therefore, is the conflict of interest between patient advocacy (providing all treatment that can possibly be of benefit—or might be perceived to be of benefit) and cost control (providing only treatment that has been demonstrated to be beneficial). And we are moving to the more serious ethical question of whether beneficial treatments will not be made available to some people because they are too expensive and there is no way to pay for them.

E. Haavi Morreim views this transition as the development of a new medical ethos (Morreim, 1995). We have come through the age of physician control and are now fast approaching the end of patient autonomy. The pendulum is set to swing back toward a middle ground of shared decision making. But the synthesis will also constitute a new stage because it will involve the economic factor that was not present before. We have arrived at a stage where payer systems now set the basic rules of the game for both physicians and patients.

Morreim sees the changing role of the patient as the key to the current stage of this revolution. At least in the immediate future, according to Morreim, patients will have to decide among various health plans with differing provisions. This will put patients more in the role of direct purchaser than ever before and will, for the first time, bring the economic factor into the physician–patient decision-making arena. Patients will have to consider what other goods they and their families are willing to forego in favor of health benefits. As Morreim explains it,

> . . . to involve patients more closely in choosing their health plans is probably the most acceptable way to bring rationing into the clinical setting. Throughout our lives we make trade-offs among the things we value, because everything we buy comes at the opportunity cost of foreclosing whatever we might instead have selected. To hold a competent adult to the consequences of his own trade-off decisions, even where this means informing him that he is not free to pursue certain options that he himself foreclosed, does not offend his autonomy.
>
> (Morreim, 1995:142)

Under this new economic medical ethos, the public in general and managed care plan members in particular need to be defended from the *free rider* problem that arises "when someone buys inadequate insurance with the expectation that, if he needs better care, everyone else will ante up and rescue him anyway" (Morreim, 1995:143). This means, Morreim explains,

> . . . that, if the patient has opted against some particular form of care that he later needs or wants, he must either pay for that care himself or go without. If his plan explicitly refuses to cover experimental care then he is not wronged if, when later his unexpected major illness can only be treated by an experimental drug, his insurer refuses to pay for it.
>
> (Moreim, 1995:145)

As an effective direction for the economics of health care, however, this model would require (as Morreim recognizes) some form of universal coverage. It makes no sense to say that patients need to exercise more responsibility for the economics of their care if some people have no choice because they cannot afford health insurance, or if there are no alternatives available, or if, as publicly insured, the government chooses for them. This direction for the health-care system also presumes a high level of economic competence on the part of consumers. Morreim suggests a variety of ways to attain this, but whether people are able to wade through the details of competing health plans (and whether the plans available really have any consequential differences) remains to be seen. At this point, people are apparently more prepared to use the political system to require MCOs to produce acceptable plans.

Mark Rodwin is less optimistic about the emergence of a new economic model for health care in the United States (Rodwin, 1993). He sees a system under pressure from the new economic incentives structure and proposes that it be repaired. In an analysis based on the concept of conflict of interest, Rodwin argues that forceful regulation is necessary to preserve the altruistic and fiduciary aspects of the current physician–patient relationship. "Regulations that restrict physicians' conflicts of interest," he concludes, "can bolster professionalism by shielding physicians from these corrupting influences. . . . Rules are sometimes needed to promote an ethos that is deeper, stronger, and more important than the rules themselves" (Rodwin, 1993:245). Rodwin's points are well taken, but his specific recommendations are subject to the limitations discussed under the points mentioned above.

George Khushf has advanced a third option focused on the development of a mid-level institutional ethos—something between Morreim's faith in economic incentives and Rodwin's efforts to shore up traditional professionalism (Khushf, 1998). At this point, however, it is not clear what kind of structure this would be or where it would acquire the power to control the forces already at play. The most likely direction for the immediate future, therefore, is still, as I have argued above, the further development of government regulation of managed care plans. We have moved from professional control of the system to economic control. If this is not morally acceptable to the public, we will move toward political control (see also Emanuel, 1995; Kassirer, 1995a, 1995b; Rimler and Morrison, 1993).

The future evolution of managed care is difficult to predict, and the picture is admittedly somewhat distorted at present by media attention to stories of people being denied care (Kurtz, 1998). There are, however, signs of positive change in managed care that deserve at least brief mention. First, there is the performance assessment and accreditation of MCOs similar to JCAHO accreditation of hospitals. The National Committee for Quality Assurance (NCQA) is a not-for-profit association of employers, consumers, providers, and plan administrators that offers a program for assessing the quality of managed care plans.

> NCQA's mission is to provide information that enables purchasers and consumers of managed health care to distinguish among plans based on quality, thereby allowing them to make more informed health care purchasing decisions. This will encourage plans to compete based on quality and value, rather than on price and provider network.
>
> (NCQA, 1998)

A second opportunity for managed care is the development of better preventive care. One of the original points of the HMO ideology was that MCOs would have an essential interest in preventive care since this would reduce later costs. Early reports indicated that MCOs offer no more preventive care than was available under indemnity insurance. But managed care is still in its infancy, with little market stability or "brand loyalty." Plans are still marketed more in terms of customer convenience and medical staff qualifications than on the basis of preventive programs. Nonetheless, the Centers for Disease Control have noted some examples of progress:

The Group Health Cooperative of Puget Sound (GHCPS) has recently summarized 20 years of its experience in primary and secondary prevention of disease [Thompson et al., 1995]. GHCPS is a large membership-governed, staff-model HMO with 486,000 members in Washington and Idaho. In 1978, GHCPS formed a Committee on Prevention and has since developed systematic approaches to programs in breast cancer screening, childhood vaccinations, influenza vaccinations for at-risk populations, smoking cessation and prevention, cholesterol screening, increased use of bicycle safety helmets by children, and detection and management of depression. . . . The programs have demonstrated a 32% decrease in late-stage breast cancer (from 1989 to 1990); a vaccination completion rate of 89% among 2-year-old children (1994); a decrease in the prevalence of smoking in adults from 25% to 17% (from 1985 to 1994); and an increase in the prevalence of use of bicycle safety helmets among children from 4% to 48%, accompanied by a 67% decrease in bicycle-related head injuries (from 1987 to 1992). Because several of the programs included community-wide policy interventions, the results may have extended beyond the GHCPS-enrolled population to the entire community.

(CDC, 1995:5)

Third, the managed care system offers the possibility of better data for medical research that will lead to improved scientific practice guidelines. The MCO information systems may be used to collect data on the effectiveness of treatment and delivery systems that have not been systematically available before. Officials of the Center for Disease Control have recognized the potential for data collection that exists in managed care systems, and MCOs themselves have formed a network of research centers to advance data collection and related research (CCDPHP, 1997).

The outcome of the transition to managed care may not be predictable at this point, but it will surely depend to a large extent on the ethical stance adopted by MCOs. The promises of the managed care revolution are evident in many of the mission statements of MCOs. The following statement from the Keystone Mercy Health Plan, a 600,000-member managed care provider in Pennsylvania, is a good example.

Keystone Mercy Health Plan exists to provide quality and accessible health care services to its members, and is characterized by a special concern for the poor and disadvantaged.

Keystone Mercy Health Plan seeks to assure that care is provided to its members by compassionate, competent professionals who are respectful of individual dignity.

Keystone Mercy Health Plan is guided by the following twelve Values as we work to achieve our Mission:

Advocacy: The promotion of justice, especially for those without power.
Care for the Poor: A special concern for and collaboration with the materially poor.
Compassion: Feeling the pain of another and comforting them.

Competence: Maintaining the skills and wisdom to do our work with excellence.

Dignity: The inherent worth of each person as gifted by the Creator.

Diversity: The fostering of an environment which values understanding, acceptance and respect of individuals in their multicultural richness.

Hospitality: Respect, inclusion, community-building and collaboration.

Leadership: The dynamic encouragement toward achieving our mission and business goals.

Quality: Excellence through continuous process improvement.

Services: Understanding the customers' needs and meeting their requirements.

Stewardship: The wise and responsible use of resources—human, financial and material—for the greater good.

Teamwork: The contribution of each person's experience, perspective and background to accomplishing the mission.

(Keystone, 1998)

This mission statement contains many of the organizational goals mentioned in Chapter 1. The implementation of ideals such as these, however, requires the development of organizations that will foster their expression. Fulfillment of these goals, whether by a single MCO or more generally by the managed care system, will be attained only if MCOs can find ways to keep cost containment and competitive market pressures from reducing the quality and availability of care. There is no place in the current healthcare system where attention to the ethical dimension of organizational decisions is more crucial at this point than in the governance and administration of managed care plans. The success or failure of this revolution depends to a large extent on whether the new system will be found morally acceptable.

This chapter has focused on the conflicts of interest generated by the managed care system. Managed care organizations also have to address most of the other issues covered elsewhere in this book–advertising, patient services, medical records, community relations, diversity, and so on. (see also Malhorta and Miller, 1996). Some MCOs are actively addressing the ethical problems generated by the system. The 1997 annual report of Harvard Pilgrim Health Care, entitled *Viewpoints: Ethics in Managed Care*, is a good example. Here is one case proposed in this report for discussion: it concerns not only the problem of approvals for procedures, but also the responsibilities of the organization for medical progress.

Case 4.1 New Medical Technology

As a member of your health plan's Technology Assessment Committee, you have the deciding vote on whether a new surgical treatment for emphysema should be covered. Unfortunately, it is not yet clear whether the procedure does patients more harm than good, and the additional costs could be significant.

The new surgical procedure is designed to reduce lung volume and alleviate some of the most debilitating symptoms of emphysema. Since your health plan doesn't cover treatments that are purely experimental, the Technology Assessment Committee is responsible for deciding when a new technology crosses the line to non-experimental.

Lung volume reduction surgery (LVRS) for emphysema, like many new medical technologies, falls in the gray area of "promising but unproven." The committee has been discussing the issue for more than three hours. Here is some of what you have learned: Lung volume reduction surgery is currently being performed at a few local hospitals that have relatively limited experience, and at a highly regarded teaching hospital with which the health plan is affiliated. At the teaching hospital, however, patients can gain access to LVRS only if they agree to participate in a clinical trial that is intended to test the effectiveness of the procedure. In the clinical trial, half [of] the patients are randomly assigned to medical treatment and half get the surgery.

To date, research and expert opinion about the effectiveness of LVRS [are] evenly divided, which is why the clinical trials are still being conducted. One surgeon on the Technology Assessment Committee argues that, despite the lack of hard evidence, she believes the new procedure enhances the quality of life for patients with advanced emphysema. Another fears that coverage will open a Pandora's Box of demand. "How about if we agree to cover it only at the teaching hospital," he suggests. That way we'll know that our patients are getting the best care, and since they'll have to participate in the clinical trial, we'll be helping find out whether LVRS really works."

Two other members discuss whether the health plan's money would be better spent on smoking prevention and cessation, and another says she's ready to throw in the towel because the legislature could pass a law requiring coverage in any case. "If we say 'no,' we'll be accused of withholding care just to save money," she says. Another member responds: "I'd rather say 'no coverage' and let our physicians seek benefit exceptions for their patients if they feel strongly enough that LVRS is the only way to go."

The debate continues: "It's unethical to spend our members' money on a procedure that is unproven and potentially harmful!" "No, its unethical to withhold coverage of a promising treatment for such a debilitating disease!"

Keeping in mind that the current research and expert opinion is evenly divided, how would you vote, and why?

(HPHC, 1997:18)

(This case is reprinted with permission of Harvard Pilgrim Health Care.)

The initial answer of many MCOs was to refuse to pay for unproven treatments. But most organizations have reconsidered their positions on this issue, in part because of competitive pressures and in part because of member appeals. In response to this case, Dr. David Eddy raised the question of the extent to which MCOs are responsible for paying for research (HPHC, 1997; see also Eddy, 1996, 1997). If a major policy of managed care is to practice by the best scientific guidelines, however, then MCOs should accept some responsibility to contribute to medical research. There is also the question of patient autonomy. If this is a treatment alternative, however weak the evidence, shouldn't a patient have the option of trying it?

CONCLUSIONS

In historical perspective, one can view the transition to managed care as a move to place control of the healthcare system in the hands of business administrators. Cost containment is necessary, but this inevitably means restricting services. Cost control measures such as prior approvals and practice guidelines, however, have created a conflict of interest for healthcare providers whose responsibilities to their MCOs may conflict with their professional judgment and traditional patient advocacy.

Efforts to overcome this conflict of interest by enhancing the professional responsibility of physicians may prove too weak to withstand the financial pressures. Legal regulations governing production incentives and informed consent laws may help. Consumer pressure for federal quality standards is more likely to be effective, however.

Although the outcome of this remarkable transition is still undecided, there are some signs of the benefits of managed care. Quality assurance through accreditation associations will help MCOs adopt higher standards of their own. Data on the effectiveness of medical procedures will improve decision making. And the benefits of early detection and better preventive care promised by better care management are beginning to appear.

The development of managed care as a healthcare delivery system raises ethical questions for all stakeholders. Patients have already felt the risk of cost containment threatening their traditional care-on-demand autonomy. Physicians have a stake in finding solutions to the conflict of interest problem—solutions that contain costs while not undermining their professional standards. And administrators, who now hold more power than ever, have a stake in making the system work: they will be praised if managed care is successful and blamed if it is not.

REFERENCES

AMA (American Medical Association), 1994, *Physician Health Plans and Networks Act of 1994*, Chicago: American Medical Association.

——, 1997, *Code of Medical Ethics: Current Opinions and Annotations*, 1996–1997 edition, Chicago: American Medical Association.

——, (Council on Ethical and Judicial Affairs), 1995, "Ethical Issues in Managed Care," *Journal of the American Medical Association*, 273(4):330–335.

Anderson, David, 1997, "Managed Care's New Ethics," *Business and Health*, 15(2):24–31.

Arras, John D., and Bonnie Steinbock, 1999, *Ethical Issues in Modern Medicine*, 5th ed., Mountain View, CA: Mayfield Publishing Company.

Biblo, Joan D., Myra J. Christopher, Linda Johnson, and Robert Lyman Potter, 1996,

"Ethical Issues in Managed Care: Guidelines for Clinicians and Recommendations to Accrediting Organizations," *Bioethics Forum*, 12: MC/1–MC/224.

CCDPHP (National Center for Chronic Disease Prevention and Health Promotion), 1997, "Tracking Managed Care Disease Prevention Efforts Through HEDIS," *Chronic Disease Notes and Reports*, 10(1):9–11.

CDC (Centers for Disease Control), 1995, "The Relationship Between Managed Care and Prevention," *Morbidity and Mortality Weekly Report*, 44(RR-14):3–6.

Chin, Marshall H., 1997, "Health Outcomes and Managed Care: Discussing the Hidden Issues," *American Journal of Managed Care*, 3:756–762.

Christensen, Kate T., 1996, "Physicians and Managed Care: Employees or Professionals?" *Bioethics Forum*, 12:17–20.

Cockerham, William C., 1997, *Medical Sociology*, Upper Saddle Ridge, NJ: Prentice-Hall.

Eddy, David, 1996, "Benefit Language: Criteria That Will Improve Quality While Reducing Costs," *Journal of the American Medical Association*, 275(8):650–658.

———, 1997, "Investigational Treatments: How Strict Should We Be?" *Journal of the American Medical Association*, 278(3):179–186.

Emanuel, Ezekiel J., 1995, "Medical Ethics in the Era of Managed Care: The Need for Institutional Structures Instead of Principles for Individual Cases," *Journal of Clinical Ethics*, 6: 335–338.

Emanuel, Ezekiel J., and Allan S. Brett, 1993, "Managed Competition and the Patient–Physician Relationship," *New England Journal of Medicine*, 329(12):879–882.

Federal Register, 1992; 57:59024–59040.

Gorman, Christine, 1998, "Playing the HMO Game," *Time*, July 13, 22–29.

Hillman, Alan L., Mark V. Pauly, and Joseph J. Kerstein, 1989, "How Do Financial Incentives Affect Physicians' Clinical Decisions and the Financial Performance of Health Maintenance Organizations?" *New England Journal of Medicine*, 321:86–92.

HPHC (Harvard Pilgrim Health Care), 1997, *Annual Report: Viewpoints: Ethics in Managed Care*, Brookline, MA: Harvard Pilgrim Health Care, Inc.

IHA (Integrated Healthcare Association), 1998, "Ethical Principles and Managed Care," http://www.iha.org/22498.htm (11/27/98).

JCAHO (Joint Commission on Accreditation of Healthcare Organizations), 1998, *Ethical Issues and Patient Rights Across the Continuum of Care*, Chicago: Joint Commission on Accreditation of Healthcare Organizations.

Kassirer, Jerome P., 1995a, "The Next Transformation in the Delivery of Health Care," *New England Journal of Medicine*, 332(1):52–53.

———, 1995b, "Managed Care and the Morality of the Marketplace," *New England Journal of Medicine*, 333(1):50–52.

Keystone (Keystone Mercy Health Plan), 1998, "Mission and Values," http://www.keystonemercyhealth.org/ (1/20/99).

Khushf, George, 1998, "A Radical Rupture in the Paradigm of Modern Medicine: Conflicts of Interest, Fiduciary Obligations, and the Scientific Ideal," *Journal of Medicine and Philosophy*, 23(1):98–122.

Kurtz, Howard, 1998, "Some Managed-Care Sagas Need Second Exam," *The Washington Post*, August 10, A01.

Lemieux-Charles, Louise, Eric M. Meslin, Ross Baker, and Peggy Leatt, 1993, "Ethical Issues Faced by Clinician/Managers in Resource-Allocation Decisions," *Hospital and Health Services Administration*, 38(2):267–285.

MacKay, K., and A. H. Moss, 1997, "To Dialyze Or Not to Dialyze: An Ethical and

Evidence-Based Approach to the Patient with Acute Renal Failure in the Intensive Care Unit," *Advances in Renal Replacement Therapy*, 4:288–296.

Malhotra, Naresh K., and Gina L. Miller, 1996, "Ethical Issues in Marketing Managed Care," *Journal of Health Care Marketing*, 16:60–65.

Margolis, Joseph, 1979, "Conflict of Interest and Conflicting Interests," in Tom L. Beauchamp and Norman E. Bowie, eds., *Ethical Theory and Business*, Englewood Cliffs, NJ: Prentice-Hall.

Morreim, E. Haavi, 1995, *Balancing Act: The New Medical Ethics of Medicine's New Economics*, Washington, DC: Georgetown University Press.

NCQA (National Committee for Quality Assurance), 1998, "National Committee for Quality Assurance: An Overview," http://www.ncqa.org/overview3.htm (4/5/98).

Rimler, George W., and Richard D. Morrison, 1993, "The Ethical Impacts of Managed Care," *Journal of Business Ethics*, 12:493–501.

RMCHE (Rocky Mountain Center for Healthcare Ethics), 1997, *Code of Ethics for Managed Care in Colorado*, Denver: Rocky Mountain Center for Healthcare Ethics.

Rodwin, Marc A., 1993, *Medicine, Money, and Morals: Physicians' Conflicts of Interest*, Oxford, UK: Oxford University Press.

S. 1890, 1998, Patients' Bill of Rights Act of 1998, http://thomas.loc.gov/ (4/4/98).

Thompson, Robert S., and Stephen H. Taplin, 1995, "Primary and Secondary Prevention Services in Clinical Practice: Twenty Years' Experience in Development, Implementation, and Evaluation," *Journal of the American Medical Association*, 273(14): 1130–1135.

Woodstock (Woodstock Theological Center), 1995, *Ethical Considerations in the Business Aspects of Health Care*, Washington, DC: Georgetown University Press.

Zoloth-Dorfman, Laurie, and Susan Rubin, 1995, "The Patient as Commodity: Managed Care and the Question of Ethics," *Journal of Clinical Ethics*, 6:339–357.

5

DIVERSITY

Race, ethnicity, and gender permeate our social interaction and our work lives. Diversity is now a major issue in organizational management and customer services. The discussion in this chapter focuses on those aspects of the subject that impinge most directly upon the normal activities of healthcare organizations: employment discrimination, sexual harassment, workplace relationships, and sexual orientation. It concludes with some comments on diversity training programs.

DISCRIMINATION

Discrimination in employment, according to the Civil Rights Act of 1964, takes place when a person is denied a position, promotion, or some other employment benefit, or is laid off, because of his or her race, color, religion, sex, or national origin. Age was added to the list as a protected class in 1967. In 1982 a separate bill was passed governing pregnancy discrimination; and in 1991 discrimination on the basis of disability was made illegal under the Americans with Disabilities Act. Individual states have added other categories, such as marital status and sexual orientation.

Discrimination persists, however. Not only is there strong evidence of stereotypical categorization of people by race and gender (Velasquez, 1998:375–387), but research on hiring practices has produced what an Urban Institute publication called "clear and convincing evidence" of outright discrimination (Fix and Strucyk, 1993). Pairs of applicants (male/female, white/African-American) equally qualified in terms of education, experience, and personal appearance have routinely been offered positions that differ widely in organizational level and compensation.

Legal guidelines for civil rights issues can be complex, but the concept is relatively straightforward. In general, the law says that adverse actions, whether in employment or public accommodation, cannot be based on a person's race, religion, sex, disability, age, or national origin. This does not mean that a person who does not do his or her job adequately cannot be discharged or that reasonable occupational qualifications cannot be considered in hiring. It means only that the decision cannot be based on, or significantly influenced by, the fact that a person is a member of one of the protected classes (female, Jewish, African-American, disabled, etc.) With respect to disabilities and religion, furthermore, employers and organizations that serve the public are expected to make a reasonable accommodation to peoples' needs.

Discrimination can be intentional, but it can also be unintentional. People can unwittingly categorize and stereotype others with respect to job performance expectations and evaluations. When this becomes a traditional practice or part of the culture of an organization, it is often referred to as *institutionalized discrimination*. In 1984, for example, Ann Hopkins brought a case in the Washington, DC, District Court charging Price Waterhouse, the giant accounting firm, with sex discrimination for denying her promotion to partnership (HBS, 1991). The court found that there was no intentional discrimination. Performance evaluations for Hopkins "were not fabricated as a pretext for discrimination," and the company had "legitimate non-discriminatory reasons" for denying her a partnership while promoting male candidates who had applied. Nonetheless, the court decided that the company's decision "was tainted by discriminatory evaluations that were the direct result of its failure to address the evident problem of sexual stereotyping," and that "discriminatory stereotyping of females was permitted to play a part" in the decision (Hopkins, 1985:1120). It was thus traditional or institutionalized, although largely unintentional, attitudes and practices that were at fault.

ETHICAL PERSPECTIVES

Equal opportunity (as distinct from affirmative action, which will be discussed later) is a strongly held American ideal. But, as sociologist Robin M. Williams found in the 1950s, public endorsement of the ideal of social equality seems to be quite compatible with individual decisions that reflect values of racism and a sense of group superiority (Williams, 1959:409, 438). The American dilemma is that the actual social value of racial superiority was and still is inconsistent with the ideal value of equality. The major thrust of Dr. Martin Luther King's appeal to the nation was to live up to its own stated values. The Civil Rights Act of 1964 was a major step in the effort to bring social practice into conformity with social ideals.

If the American ideal is inconsistent with actual social practice on this score, however, our major ethical perspectives are not ambivalent at all. Over and above its illegality, discrimination is morally wrong from a utilitarian perspective because judging people on the basis of stereotypes does not maximize benefit to them personally or to society in general. When discrimination takes place in employment, people who could potentially do the job better and thereby add to the common good are summarily excluded because of their race, gender, disability, or other characteristics irrelevant to job performance. Social benefit can be maximized only by distributing jobs on the basis of abilities.

From the rational perspective, people should also be judged on the basis of their merits. Characteristics over which one has little or no control and which are not relevant to one's work performance have no place in evaluations of one's worth in the context of employment, just as they have no place in the context of service in public places of business or in renting or purchasing property. If one expects his or her integrity as a person to be respected, it is irrational to deny similar respect to others. From most utilitarian and rational perspectives, furthermore, discrimination based on sexual orientation, marital status, political ideology, or any other irrelevant status would be equally unethical, regardless of whether these characteristics are included in a list of legally protected classes.

While the vast majority of idealist traditions hold that individuals should not be judged on the basis of irrelevant characteristics, it must be said that there is considerable variation among these ethical perspectives. Some religious groups hold that race and gender are indeed relevant with respect to social or civic roles as well as with respect to family responsibilities. Both in the ancient world and in early American tradition, religiously based as it was, those who were thought to be created equal did not include women or slaves. And today many religious idealists consider gender and sexual orientation to be relevant to social decisions as well as to personal or private lifestyles. The extent to which the civil rights movement has been motivated by religious ideals must not be neglected, however, nor should the social influence of the strong human rights positions adopted many religious organizations be underestimated.

Regardless of the basis of their theoretical perspective, most moral philosophers use the language of human rights to express their ethical commitments in this area, although they do so with slightly different meanings. Utilitarian theorists who see the use of rules as the best way to maximize welfare are inclined to list the right to equal treatment regardless of race, gender, ethnicity, religion, disability, and so on as basic rules and to support laws that embody these rules. Rationalists who view respect for individuals as the most basic imperative of the moral law often use the language of human rights to formulate this belief. And moral theologians often hold that respect for human rights is implicit in God's will for social life. So there is a certain amount of overlap in terminology here and a general consensus at the level of principles despite theoretical differences with respect to the underlying justification.

From a stakeholder perspective, it should be clear that employees and prospective employees have an interest in being considered on their own merits. There are, nevertheless, pressures from the other side; people often feel that they have a claim because of prior service (seniority) or special relations (prior commitments). Hiring and promotion on the basis of connections can, however, have a detrimental effect on other employees who may resent a corporate culture that involves favoritism. Equal opportunity is good business on at least two counts: finding the best person for the job and promoting confidence in the fairness of organizational decisions.

Antidiscrimination principles are found in many healthcare organizational mission statements, particularly those of institutions with religious affiliations.

> We respect patients' different needs in our multicultural and multilingual community.
>
> (St. Joseph's Hospital, 1998)

> . . . we have a duty toward God and our neighbor in justice and charity; therefore everyone who approaches us for care, regardless of race, creed, nationality, age, sex, handicap, or economic status, is entitled to share in the fruits of our ministry.
>
> (St. Francis, 1999)

If mission statements are taken seriously, they can focus attention on what can be done to develop organizational procedures that will help prevent the occurrence of discrimination. Regular review of hiring and promotion practices to ensure equal opportunity is important. Clear guidelines for job descriptions and performance evaluations may give managers a more objective sense of their task and a stronger capacity to resist pressures from the (quite normal) human tendency to "look out for one's own" and to underestimate the skills and abilities of others.

While there would appear to be consensus among ethical perspectives concerning most types of discrimination, practical problems for healthcare managers persist. Consider the following dilemma.

Case 5.1 Customer Preference

A long-term care subdivision of a small regional hospital has 90 intermediate-care beds and 20 skilled-care beds. It employs a typical staff of nurses, aides, and maintenance people. Following an incident in which a patient and her family had refused care from the African-American nurse on duty, the organization was sued for discrimination. Kendra Wilson, a nurse on one 30-bed wing, had complained to the director that this was the third time in two years that she had been shifted to a different unit because a patient had refused to have an African-American nurse. The director simply said that there was nothing she could do: the patient's family had made the request. She tried to talk them out of it, but they insisted that it was upsetting to their mother to have a black person take care of her. Since this was the only single room available at the time, the only way to solve the problem was to transfer Wilson to another unit. The director apologized, saying that Wilson was indeed one of their most competent nurses, but insisted that she had no choice. "It is really for your own good," she said. "I wouldn't want you to be embarrassed by this family."

The legal notice came in the form of a letter from the state's Human Rights Commission notifying the hospital that a complaint had been filed by Ms. Wilson. The Commission requested the following information: Had Wilson indeed been transferred because of this customer's preference? What percentage of clients and staff were African-American? Was it the policy of the facility to make staff transfers on the basis of race?

The nursing home director contacted the hospital's lawyer for advice. She was told to reply that acceding to her patients' wishes was a business necessity for the nursing home, that other staff members were sometimes reassigned at the request of patients (which was quite true), and that this was thus not a matter of discrimination on the basis of race. "Just tell the Human Rights people that it is your normal practice to accommodate patients' wishes," the lawyer said, "not a matter of race."

This case raises many questions. Is the lawyer's response truthful? Should Wilson have been reassigned? Is accommodating a client's prejudices any more justifiable than acting on one's own prejudices? If Wilson had not been reassigned, what should the family have been told? Should this incident have any effect on the recruitment of nurses in the future? Does the argument that this was a business necessity constitute a legal defense?

Two problems in particular are worth special consideration here. The first is a practical issue: what does one do in the immediate situation when an action is clearly contrary to the ethical standards of the organization but a patient's care requires it? Suppose, for example, that the patient in question had shouted at Wilson, refused to allow Wilson to touch her, or even thrown something at her when she entered the room. The patient would still have to be cared for at the nursing home until other arrangements could be made. The care that this patient requires, regardless of her attitude, is a moral responsibility based on the facility's prior commitment to her family that cannot simply be ignored. Acceding to the patient's demands by recognizing her need for care could only be justified, however, in the context of addressing the larger issue in a way that will ultimately uphold the diversity policy of the organization. In fact, Wilson was primarily interested in forcing the organization to take a stand on the issue that was consistent with its own stated policy. She did not want to deny care to anyone, regardless of his or her racist attitude. The case demonstrates, however, that organizations need to address issues effectively and in a timely manner rather than with makeshift solutions that just put the problem off until the next occurrence. Contrary to the paternalistic attitude of the director toward her, Wilson was not as offended by the racist opinions of the patient as by the refusal of the nursing home to deal with the issue in a manner that was consistent with its mission statement. To her, the persistence of the makeshift solution, with no effort to solve or prevent the problem in the future, indicated that the organization was itself racist despite its claim to the contrary.

The second, and larger, issue here is more hypothetical but just as practical. Would the situation be the same if this were a case of gender discrimination? For example, what if an elderly nun did not want to be cared for by a male nurse? Should the nurse be reassigned? Is gender discrimination somehow different from racial discrimination? This may be more of a question of personal modesty than gender discrimination. Or it might even be related to the nun's religious vows. People will surely disagree about this matter, but I sense a difference here. If the nun was comfortable with the care of the male nurse other than for matters of personal hygiene, it could be considered a question of modesty rather than one of gender bias.

DEALING WITH DIVERSITY: ACCOMMODATION VERSUS INTEGRITY

Beyond compliance with civil rights laws, there is a wide range of clinical and organizational problems that entail conflicts between service to clients and the ideals of the organization. Basically these issues involve patients' requests for services (or the withholding or withdrawal of treatment) that the physician and the organization are reluctant to give because of their ethical commitments. The request for an abortion in a Roman Catholic hospital is an obvious example.

The dilemma here can be formulated as a conflict between values. On the one hand there is a commitment to diversity, which would require an institution or an individual to accommodate the religious beliefs of patients. Thus adult, competent Jehovah's Witnesses are normally allowed to refuse blood transfusions. Physicians often make adjustments in what they might see as physiologically the best plan of care in order to accommodate these patients. There may, of course, be times when a surgeon might refuse to undertake a certain operation without the use of blood replacement, but this refusal is based on medical inadvisability, not on moral or religious beliefs or institutional policy. In any case, accommodating individual requests is clearly a goal for healthcare providers and organizations. The case of L'Hôpital St. Jean Baptiste Missionaire at the end of this chapter poses some questions about the limits of this type of accommodation.

On the other side of the issue of diversity, and sometimes at odds with the value of accommodation, is the moral integrity of the institution. Some individuals and organizations, for example, are morally opposed to withholding or withdrawing nutrition and hydration from terminal patients. Others are opposed to the use of certain techniques to assist reproduction. A Jewish nursing home, in a case study in the *Hastings Center Report*, prohibited nonkosher food even though only 10% of its residents were observant Orthodox Jews (Boyle and Hanson, 1993). For these institutions it is a matter of principle. Even though they may be committed to accommodating people's wishes, accommodation has its limits.

So accommodation and integrity can be at odds both individually and in organizational policy. Let me continue this discussion with an example related to the question of whether a Roman Catholic hospital should offer antipregnancy prophylaxis to a rape victim. Erich Loewy has argued that, as a member of a hospital ethics committee at a Catholic hospital, he should not be expected to adopt the religious perspective or the ethical principles of the institution. The ethics committee was asked to write a policy addressing services to rape victims, but was told that the policy had to conform to the church's teachings as interpreted by the local bishop. This put Loewy in a position he clearly resented. A policy of sending rape victims to another hospital or an off-campus physician was not, in his view, an acceptable option from a clinical perspective. Nor was advising physicians to write prescriptions for patients to be filled elsewhere an acceptable option since technically this would have violated hospital policy. Loewy thus found himself on an ethics committee that was being told what to do in no uncertain terms, and he could see no solution to the problem. Finding the situation intolerable, he concluded that "when individual morality conflicts with institutional policy, members of ethics committees should be free to voice and act upon their opinions rather than be expected to follow rigid preestablished and ordained dogma" (Loewy, 1994:584).

Apart from his personal involvement, Loewy's position on the organizational issue was that since the hospital serves a community that includes non-Catholics, it must accommodate these patients, especially in such crucial situations as rape. "When hospitals are dedicated to caring for the public at large and when they receive public funds, they must try to adjust their services and actions to the public need" (583–584). According to Loewy, this conclusion is implied in the nature of ethics committees themselves:

> Virtually all persons who have had a hand in shaping the concept of ethics committees in this country accept the principle that the individuals making up the committee should represent different interests, backgrounds, and viewpoints. In other words, ethics committees are intended mainly to represent the interests of the communities they serve.
>
> (Loewy, 1994:578)

While the adequacy of medical services (accommodating the needs of the patient) is a clinical question in part, the nature and mandate of the committee itself are organizational issues involving the integrity of the institution in terms of its mission. And much as I appreciate the dilemma in which Loewy found himself, I think his conclusion is wrong. If we expect institutions to act responsibly as moral agents, and to adopt and implement institutional goals, we have to be prepared to accept the concept of institutional integrity, that is, the idea that its ethical principles are essential to its mission. We cannot expect an organization to overlook its principles and commitments in order to accommodate all patients' requests or community expectations (Orr, 1995; Siegel, 1995).

As a clinical issue, the rape victim should certainly be offered whatever treatment is medically appropriate. But Loewy addressed this issue on the organizational level, asking whether an ethics committee should be subject to the implications of the overall mission of the institution. I believe it should, so some arrangement other than asking the institution to compromise its principles will have to be found. I hasten to add, however, that members of ethics committees must act according to their own beliefs and, in cases like this, register their dissent.

This is not an easy problem. In a 1984 letter to the *New England Journal of Medicine*, Dr. John Goldenring argued that since rape is an emergency situation, Catholic hospitals should be required to offer prophylactic treatment:

> Church hospitals have a right to their own moral convictions, but insofar as they act as public emergency facilities, they must provide rape victims who do not subscribe to the same moral code the right to choose immediate anti-pregnancy prophylaxis, as is indicated for optimal medical care.
>
> (Goldenring, 1984:1637)

This rationale could be persuasive, depending on how critical the emergency is and how readily available other providers are. (Roman Catholic theology allows exceptions to dogma in certain cases, but I leave this for theological debate.) In Loewy's scenario, however, other providers were readily available and the treatment to avoid pregnancy can be administered up to 72 hours after the assault. So I would still say that an institution should not be expected to compromise its own integrity unless there is no alternative. This could happen in some emergency situations involving reproductive services in Catholic hospitals and non-Catholic emergency patients or even in a (hypothetical) Jehovah's Witness hospital that might be required to give blood to a non-Witness in a life-threatening situation.

In this conflict between accommodation of a diverse mix of patients and institutional integrity, however, it would be reasonable to draw the line at the refusal of a Catholic hospital to inform a rape victim of the availability of antipregnancy treatment elsewhere. This is the point at which accommodation must be given priority. The patient needs to know what alternatives are available in order to be able to live by *her* moral principles, even if the treatment is not available at the institution at which she finds herself. Informing the patient of her options is a matter of informed consent—a principle that requires that all alternatives be disclosed (see Chapter 11). So at this point the tables turn, and it is the integrity of the patient, not the institution, that is paramount; the institution could refuse to compromise its own principles only by directly violating the moral rights of the patient. The Catholic hospital has a duty to inform the rape victim—even a Catholic—of all available treatment options. I would also say that at a nonsectarian hospital interested in accommodating people of all faiths, a physician ought to inform a Catholic rape victim of her right to have the advice of a Catholic priest before deciding on the antipregnancy prophylactic treatment. Conflicts among basic values often require a certainly flexibility in drawing the line (Boozang, 1996). In the United States, pacifists have the right not to be drafted into military service: the country accommodates their moral belief to this extent. But pacifists do not have a right to refuse to pay taxes that will be used to build nuclear weapons, since this presumably is a matter of national security.

The conflict between personal values and institutional integrity came to the fore in a 1986 New Jersey case in which a hospital was forced, contrary to its policy, to honor a patient's wish to refuse artificial nutrition and hydration (Requena, 1986). In this case, the patient refused transfer to another institution that would accommodate her wishes. The court nonetheless ordered the hospital not to discharge her and to treat her as she requested. This conclusion, Stephen Wear has argued, essentially denied the institutional integrity of the organization (Wear, 1991). Wear is right; we cannot expect institutions to develop a strong mission and foster an atmosphere of moral integrity if courts are going to order them to set their beliefs aside for the desires of a patient when a clear alternative is available. There are genuine dilemmas in which principles must be compromised, but this case appears to have been decided by setting the value of institutional integrity at naught.

Efforts to accommodate individual beliefs can also raise problems of distributive justice. In 1995, the *Hastings Center Report* carried a case study of a young Jehovah's Witness who refused transfusion before major surgery, knowing that she might die (Post and Fleck, 1995). When transfusion did become necessary, her life was saved by a very expensive ($100,000) and radical procedure of putting her in a chemical coma for two weeks to slow down her life processes. The opinions of the commentators on this case differed. Stephen Post argued that the hospital should not have paid for this extraordinary care required only because of the patient's religious beliefs. The right of informed consent (i.e., the refusal of blood) does not entail a positive entitlement to community resources. People with such beliefs should take financial responsibility for the consequences. Leonard Fleck, on the other hand, argued that since healthcare organizations do care for people who foolishly endanger their own health in other ways, and usually offer this care at their own expense, it would be inconsistent to refuse treatment here.

SEXUAL HARASSMENT

Since 1984 antidiscrimination laws have also covered sexual harassment (Vinson, 1986). *Quid pro quo sexual harassment* is defined as unwelcome language and actions of a sexual nature that affect an employee's terms or conditions of employment such as pay, promotion, benefits, or job assignments. An organization can be held legally liable for the actions of a manager, as opposed to those of coworkers, even if the organization did not know of those actions, since managers are presumed to be direct agents of organizations. A *sexually hostile environment*, on the other hand, is a situation in which comments or actions of a sexual nature interfere with the ability of an employee to perform of his or her job. These could be the words or actions of a coworker, a patient, a salesperson, or an independent physician working in a hospital, as well as those of a supervisor. The organization can be held legally liable for permitting a sexually hostile environment if an employee's superiors knew or should have known about the situation and failed to take corrective action. Same-sex sexual harassment, which is possible irrespective of the sexual orientation of either party, is now clearly covered by civil rights laws as well (Oncale, 1998).

Sexual harassment is certainly one area where "an ounce of prevention is worth a pound of cure." Healthcare organizations necessarily include people who have power and influence. A real danger in such organizations is that people will be tempted to misuse that power for their own sexual gratification unless the culture clearly indicates to them that it is inappropriate and will not be tolerated. Posting sexual harassment policies that inform employees and patients of their rights may appear to be an admission that problems exist, especially in organizations where it is widely known who the troublesome people are. But posting policies, in addition to reducing the organization's legal risk, lets less powerful people know that they do not have to tolerate inappropriate behavior. Speaking personally to offenders or potential offenders, in fact, is often easier than one might think since offenders generally know quite well that what they are doing is wrong.

Case 5.2 Third-Party Harassment

Whether a third party can claim that an environment is sexually hostile if a consensual sexual relationship in the workplace leads to favoritism for a coworker is an interesting question. Consider the following case. The Admitting Service at Adams County Medical Center (ACMC), a private, nonprofit institution, employs eight people: the director, two assistants, and five clerks. The assistants act as senior admitting clerks. Shortly after Sally Crawford was hired as an admitting clerk, she met Bill Kramer from the ACMC Office of the General Counsel. Kramer was routinely assigned to answer questions for the Admitting Service and was a close friend of the Admitting Service Director, Frank Morreschi. Sally and Bill struck up a friendship that developed into an intimate relationship—or so it seemed. (He was married and had a teenage daughter.) Bill and Sally ate lunch together, often left work together, and would sometimes, as one of the other clerks said, "disappear into the small staff room and lock the door for ten minutes or so." On one occasion, Bill and Sally attended an out-of-state conference on hospital admitting procedures together.

Most people in the office were aware of this relationship, but it did not seem to affect the daily routine. It wasn't the first office romance they had seen and probably wouldn't be the last. The only complaint anyone had was that after her first four months at ACMC, Sally was always assigned to the morning shift (7 A.M. to 3 P.M.), while other staff members had to rotate to cover the evening hours (11 A.M. to 7 P.M.).

The problem developed when one of the assistant directors resigned and Sally got the promotion. This led to a complaint of sexual harassment by two of the other admitting clerks. They did not allege that they had been harassed themselves, but rather that the relationship between Bill and Sally had created, for them, a discriminatory, sexually hostile environment. Sally was favored, they said, because she was "fooling around" with one of the hospital's lawyers. They both claimed that Bill Kramer had made advances to them previously, which they had refused. They did not consider his advances to be sexual harassment, but now, they said, they were victims of retaliation since Sally had received a promotion. They would have been considered for the promotion, they said, if they had accepted Bill's advances.

The law is not settled on this point. While some courts have held that individuals cannot claim discrimination on the basis of other people's relationships, other courts have found that they can. In this case, however, the charge of retaliation may be more serious since it is based on a claim regarding sexual approaches to the employees making the complaint. The approaches themselves may not have constituted harassment, but the loss of a job opportunity later could be considered disparate treatment based on a refusal of unwanted sexual behavior. Favoritism based on personal relationships is surely unethical since it denies equality of opportunity to other employees, but this situation is perhaps best treated managerially as a question of a conflict of interest.

PERSONAL RELATIONSHIPS IN THE WORKPLACE

Personal relationships (i.e., intimate or romantic relationships) in the workplace are, in one important respect, the exact opposite of sexual harassment. Both involve sexuality, but sexual harassment is unwanted or unwelcome sexual attention and is illegal; workplace relationships are intentional and, barring unusual circumstances, are quite legal (BNA, 1988). Workplace romance is, by definition, a matter of mutual consent.

The conventional wisdom until the 1980s was that "business and social life don't mix." Commentators and management consultants are still fond of quoting Margaret Mead's opinion that workplace relationships should be taboo (Mead, 1978). This opinion is striking not only for its absolute prohibition of such relationships, but also because Mead was certainly not known for her puritanical attitudes. Actually, the commentators have misinterpreted Mead to a certain extent. Her remarks were made in a discussion of sexual harassment, not consensual relationships. Mead, in fact, was herself involved in personal relationships at work. She met two of her three husbands on the job and was involved in an intimate relationship with a third colleague.

The pre-1980s conventional wisdom is reflected in a *Harvard Business Review* article by Senior Editor Eliza Collins (1983). Collins stated that the individuals involved in workplace relationships should be advised to seek professional help and that "either the person least essential to the company or both have to go." The conventional wisdom was challenged in the 1980s, however, in a number of studies that took a more tolerant attitude, often suggesting that personal relationships in the workplace should be managed properly rather than strictly forbidden (Jamison, 1983; Mainiero, 1989).

Public opinion and business practices have changed as well. A 1988 poll conducted by the Gallup Organization using a random sample found that 47% of the sample approved "of unmarried co-workers having an intimate relationship" (*Newsweek*, Feb. 15, 1988). A 1991 survey conducted by the Society for Human Resource Management (SHRM, 1991) found that 92.4% of the organizations represented by the nearly 1500 respondents had no policy about coworker relationships. Only 1.5% of the organizations forbade dating within the organization, 28.1% permitted but discouraged such relationships, and 70.3% simply accepted them.

One reason for the greater tolerance of workplace relationships in recent years may be that employers are becoming more sensitive to the rights of employees as individuals. As management has assumed a more relaxed, cooperative style, superiors have become more sensitive to subordinates as individuals. Tolerance is thus to some extent simply a consequence of managers' reluctance to intrude into the private lives of workers. Ethically, therefore, this must be considered as part of the expanding scope of workers' rights (see Chapter 10). Intimacy is a natural human need. Friendly relations in the workplace lead to friendships outside the workplace, and this in turn can lead to romantic involvement. Workplaces bring together people with similar backgrounds, similar education, and similar interests. It would be unusual if work colleagues with such similarities, who also share extensive work experiences, were not attracted to one another. Organizations that promote personal relationships through workplace picnics, parties, exercise facilities, and team sports, furthermore, cannot avoid promoting intimate relationships. Nowhere is this more true than in healthcare organizations. Health care requires close teamwork, including emotional involvement among people with similar educational levels, interests, and life goals. If people spend most of their waking hours at work, this setting tends to be the only place to fulfill the need for intimacy, as well as the various needs (money, respect, creativity) associated with the work itself. Work has become the most natural place to meet compatible, attractive people with similar interests. Ethical analysis cannot ignore social realities.

However, while the development of personal relationships in the workplace may be natural for the individuals involved, it can have undesirable consequences for the organization. Problems associated with workplace relationships range from office gossip to major abuses of power and misuse of funds. Gossip itself may be a form of complaint that all is not well in the workplace. Distractions can interfere with patient care; people may seek or avoid contact with others because of outside relationships that have nothing to do with their professional duties.

If the consequences of workplace relationships pose problems for the organization, then addressing these consequences is the appropriate organizational response. It is the job performance of the individuals involved that is at issue, not the relationship itself. An organization can reasonably expect workplace relationships not to interfere with performance (Colby, 1991). The ethical response, therefore, is to treat the issue as a matter of productivity. This is the best strategy when workplace issues involve questions of civil rights. Decisions based on productivity rather than on status are more likely to be legally correct and managerially effective. The same is true of matters that can be considered workers' rights.

Serious problems with workplace relationships, furthermore, may occur when the relationship is between a superior and a subordinate. In the 1991 SHRM survey, 48 respondents (3%) offered the unsolicited opinion that the real issue is not workplace relationships but superior-subordinate relationships. There is always a risk to the organization if a supervisor's judgment is clouded by favoritism. And even if favoritism is avoided, actions may easily be perceived as involving favoritism by coworkers and can be bad for morale (Anderson and Fisher, 1991; Anderson and Hunsaker, 1985). Even without any deterioration in performance, therefore, a workplace relationship between a superior and a subordinate may constitute a conflict of interest because it holds the potential for compromising company loyalty and professional decision making. A conflict of interest is not in itself an action with adverse consequences, but it involves the risk of adverse consequences by placing a person in a position in which he or she is tempted or could be coerced into performing a harmful act. It would be quite reasonable, therefore, for an organization to have a general policy prohibiting workplace relationships between superiors and subordinates.

SEXUAL ORIENTATION

Sexual orientation is included in civil rights protections in some states. Contrary to public opinion, however, it is legal in most states and under federal law for a person to be refused employment, denied promotion, or fired because of his or her sexual orientation. From a utilitarian perspective, discrimination on the basis of sexual orientation denies the organization the possible benefit of talented employees. And from a rational perspective, it denies equality of opportunity to gay and lesbian members of the community. But many religious people believe that gay and lesbian sexual orientations and activities are sinful or intolerable. On the social level, therefore, we face the ethical question of whether our civil society will continue to uphold its traditional moral limits, or whether it will expand them to include sexual orientations that have previously been excluded.

As a practical matter of employment policy, healthcare organizations face two questions: whether to extend nondiscrimination employment protections to gay and lesbian people and whether to include gay and lesbian partners in employment benefits programs.

Organizational policy and procedures handbooks, as well as organizational codes and mission statements, typically contain statements affirming that the organization is an equal opportunity employer. But they do not often state explicitly that sexual orientation is included as a status protected from discrimination. Arguments against inclusion are that such a statement might be offensive to some patients and staff members or to community groups and that its inclusion would involve the added legal risk of going beyond what state law requires. Arguments in favor of inclusiveness are that it is a matter of equal opportunity since a person's sexual orientation is irrelevant to his or her job performance, and that gay and lesbian people deserve to be treated as fully participating members of the community. Since explicit inclusion in institutional policy would not require other individuals to change any of their beliefs, it seems to me that the arguments for the inclusion of sexual orientation in organizational equal opportunity policies should prevail ethically. While cultural pressure to the contrary may be strong, the minority of gay and lesbian people, whose lives are less than full because they have to live under an oppressive "don't ask, don't tell" policy, would seem to have the greatest stake in the matter even though they are often socially inhibited from advancing their interests publicly. Explicit inclusion in equal opportunity protections policies sends a strong message to an important segment of our society.

The inclusion of same-sex domestic partners in organizational benefits programs is a related issue. Since the mid-1990s, an increasing number of organizations have expanded their employee benefits programs to include domestic partner benefits. According to a report by the National Lesbian and Gay Journalists Association, "the number of U.S. employers providing domestic partner benefits grew from approximately five in 1989 to 230 in 1995 and to more than 500 at the beginning of 1997" (NLGJA, 1997). This group includes a number of healthcare organizations (Kaiser Medical Group, Beth Israel Medical Center, Blue Cross/Blue Shield in Massachusetts and New Hampshire, Montefiore Medical Center, Glaxo Wellcome, Group Health, Aetna Insurance), as well as over 50 city and county governments and 23 Fortune 500 companies.

The financial costs of extending benefits to same-sex domestic partners are surprisingly low, typically less than 0.5 percent of medical benefits expenses, according to the National Lesbian and Gay Journalists Association (NLGJA, 1997). Enrollment has not been as high as was originally predicted, perhaps because gay and lesbian workers are reluctant to identify themselves or because many same-sex domestic partners are employed and covered separately. Insurance companies, which had originally added a surcharge for such coverage, have since dropped the requirement. Expenses are considerably higher if opposite-sex domestic partners are included, but many companies have refused to take this further step since heterosexual partners can obtain benefits by getting married if they wish. Legal attempts to obtain benefits for nonmarried heterosexual couples have not been successful.

AFFIRMATIVE ACTION

Affirmative action is an especially controversial and complex issue. The discussion here represents only a few aspects of the question that are important for healthcare organizations. At the outset, it is helpful to be clear about the distinction between civil rights laws, which ensure equal opportunity and are widely supported by public opinion in the United States, and affirmative action programs, which give preferences to women and minorities and have been the subject of considerable public controversy.

Affirmative action is complex because federal requirements and court decisions have been inconsistent and confusing. Basically, any organization that has a contract with the federal government is required to have an affirmative action program. The program must contain three elements: First, the organization does a detailed study of the representation of women and minorities in each of its major job classifications to see whether there are fewer women and minorities at each level than would be expected given the availability of qualified applicants in the recruitment area. Second, if the affirmative action study shows that women and minorities are underrepresented in the workforce, the organization must set goals and a timetable for correcting the imbalance. Third, the organization must appoint an affirmative action officer to coordinate efforts to recruit women and minorities until the goals of the plan are met (OFCCP, 1984).

Federal policies, furthermore, do not establish quotas and have never required that unqualified or less qualified women and minorities be given preference over more qualified applicants (OFCCP, 1984). Affirmative action laws require only that preference be given to minorities and women when candidates are *equally* qualified. Individuals, of course, are never exactly equal, and judgment is required to assess abilities relevant to the essential functions of a position from test scores, education, and experience. In healthcare organizations, the fact that a candidate would bring diversity to a workforce can itself be a desirable qualification if having a workforce that reflects the diversity of the community or the clientele is a goal of the organization.

The legal history of affirmative action, however, is not so straightforward. While the Supreme Court approved affirmative action in hiring, for example, it did not approve it for layoffs, stating that existing seniority commitments must be honored unless the seniority system was itself a product of prior discrimination. In these instances, however, discrimination must be judged on an individual basis rather than as having an effect on a class of people, which is the principle used in hiring. The Court has also been unclear about which aspects of its decisions are mandatory and which are nonbinding advisory statements, and has at times required proof of intent while elsewhere relying only on consequences. The upshot, according to Manuel Velasquez of Santa Clara University, is that

> the Supreme Court has vacillated on the constitutionality of affirmative action programs. Depending on the period in question, the issue at stake, and the makeup of the Court, it has tended both to support and to undermine affirmative action programs. Like the public itself, which remains deeply divided on the issue, the Supreme Court has had trouble making up its mind whether to support or attack these programs.
>
> (Velasquez, 1998:399)

As recognized in a 1995 statement by the American College of Healthcare Executives, however, affirmative action is now much more a question of institutional policy than of legal compliance (ACHE, 1995). If a healthcare organization emphasizes the goal of having its workforce reflect the diversity of its community, by making this a part of its mission statement and through leadership that gives serious consideration to minority groups in employment and promotion decisions, then the attention of those responsible for achieving these goals can be directed to implementation rather than to debates about affirmative action in the past.

DIVERSITY PROGRAMS

Increasingly, healthcare organizations, along with other businesses, have realized that diversity issues are a legitimate subject of their concern. First, health care is a major social institution and thus a natural stage on which social issues are played out. Where would diversity be more important than in a social service industry based on close personal interaction between professionals, staff members, and the people they serve (Carnevale and Stone, 1995)? Second, attention to diversity is good business: building and maintaining a diversity-friendly culture in the workplace enhances productivity in terms of client services. It is a matter of attracting and retaining good employees, improving organizational effectiveness, and relating to target populations (Capowski, 1996).

As an ethical ideal, diversity goes beyond toleration. While *antidiscrimination* and *affirmative action* may refer to behavior, *diversity* extends to attitudes, feelings, and beliefs. It develops when people begin to realize the fullness of life or personal satisfaction and enrichment that come from knowing and working with others who are quite different from themselves. This is why people speak of diversity as being valued, not just tolerated. As the sociologist Emile Durkheim pointed out, ethics is not just a set of rules or principles to be followed; it is an ideal that attracts and calls us to a better life (Durkheim, 1906).

The ethical basis for an organizational diversity program in health care should be obvious. An institutional mission statement will surely include the goal of serving all people, regardless of their race, gender, ethnicity, and so on. Besides, the whole point of stakeholder analysis is to be inclusive. In American society today diversity is simply a reality (Loden, 1996). In our largest cities, what were formerly minority groups now constitute the majority and less than 20% of the new people now entering the workforce are white males.

Diversity programs take a wide variety of forms, and an equally wide range of consultants and materials are available (AIMD, 1998; DTG, 1998; ICD, 1996). It is especially important, however, that the approach be adapted to the existing corporate culture and the specific needs of the organization. A program developed locally may have advantages that a predesigned or standardized program would not have and may be more effective for having been developed by its own participants. Diversity is now more than just a matter of gender and racial justice. As R. Roosevelt Thomas, Jr. (1991:10) has said, "Diversity . . . extends to age, personal and corporate background, education, function and personality . . . it includes lifestyle, sexual preference, geographic origin, tenure with the organization, exempt or nonexempt status and management or nonmanagement." Perhaps the most common and egregious error companies make, according to Genevieve Capowski (1996:17), "is to think of diversity in terms of everyone except white heterosexual males."

SERVING A DIVERSE POPULATION

Much has been written about patients' need for sensitivity to their cultural differences. JCAHO standards specifically address the issue of language and the need for interpretation services: "The medical staff, in collaboration with others, develops a formal process to guide and support the . . . availability of translation services when appropriate" (JCAHO, 1996:RI-9). Interpretation, however, is a difficult matter and should not be left to staff members who happen to speak the language or to family members. Cultural sensitivity, furthermore, goes beyond language. Religious differences are important, as are cultural traditions. In areas where healthcare organizations serve culturally diverse communities, constant planning and staff and professional training are needed. And there are times when a clinical ethics committee may be helpful in negotiating a plan of care that will take patients' values and beliefs into account.

A good illustration of cultural awareness in a clinical setting was published by Multicultural Health Care Solutions, a Texas healthcare consulting group specializing in intercultural provider–patient and provider–family interaction (MHCS, 1999). In this case, a simply dressed Southeast Asian couple brings their son in to have a physical exam and be immunized according to school policy. The chart indicates that they are Cambodian. A 6 foot 4 inch African-American male physician comes into the exam room, notices that they seem a little shy or nervous, and tries to put them at ease by being as friendly and relaxed as possible. He greets them with a big smile and shakes the father's hand robustly. He gets down on the little boy's level, says "Hi!" and ruffles his hair. No one says a word. The mother is staring at the floor; the child is staring at the floor. The physician starts to wonder if they're afraid because he is black but decides to keep being as friendly as possible. When the physician listens to the child's lungs, he discovers some alarming marks on his back. They are reddish bruises in a stripe pattern, and look as if they were made with a straight stick such as a broom handle. Now the family's unresponsiveness makes sense to him; he suspects the parents have been beating the child and don't want anyone to know. He wonders whether to call in a report to the child protective service or try to work it out privately with the family.

The authors analyzed this case as follows:

> *Awareness:* In this case study, a culturally aware provider might realize that the behavior of the family is representative of a different style of polite communication, rather than interpreting it as attitude or affect. Southeast Asians generally prefer a reserved and formal style of communication, with a great deal less direct eye contact than the mainstream American is accustomed to. The family's initial behavior is not shy or nervous, it's polite and normal, by their culture.
>
> *Knowledge:* Most Asians, including Cambodians, are very uncomfortable with social touching. A handshake, such as the physician gave to the father, is acceptable but not particularly enjoyable, especially a vigorous one. A limp handshake from an Asian, again, does not imply affect or a "weak personality"! Touching the head, even of children, can be quite offensive . . . as frightening for that person as if the physician drew a skull and crossbones on an American child's head. Unfortunately, the physician's attempts to be friendly (by touching, smiling broadly, speaking energetically) probably just made the family uncomfortable.

The marks on the child's back were the result of "coining," a common traditional Asian health practice. A coin is rubbed vigorously on the skin to release "bad wind." (The symptoms of "bad wind" are muscle ache, headache, cough, and/or sore throat—all rather "everyday" symptoms; thus coining is not an infrequent practice among those who do practice it.) This practice is no more exotic or threatening to traditional Asians than taking aspirin or milk of magnesia is to traditional Americans.

Emotions: Possible emotions in this case are the physician's tension as he keeps wondering if he's doing the right thing, culturally speaking; possible resentment on the part of the physician if he attributes the family's lack of response to racism; the parents' bewilderment at not knowing how the health care system works or what is supposed to happen next; the family's being overwhelmed by the physician's "friendliness," which they perceive as intense; and the family's embarrassment and shock when the physician ruffles the son's head.

Skills: Some skills that would be useful for the provider in this case are a more formal and low-key style of greeting, using Mr./Mrs. + name, speaking quietly and slowly, not smiling excessively, and not touching; focusing on the parents sufficiently first; taking the necessary time to establish rapport appropriately through formal self-introduction, small talk, genuinely concerned inquiry about the boy's health, and general history-taking before attempting any exam, procedure, etc. For example, in this case, the physician, after establishing rapport, could have finished the exam, making a mental note of the bruises, then calmly asked the parents if they use any home remedies for minor illnesses.

(MHCS, 1999)

The development of cultural awareness and diversity programs illustrates the need for close cooperation between a clinical ethics committee and administrators. While the clinical ethics committee might design educational programs to address cultural awareness in serving patients, it is the responsibility of administrators to promote these programs as well as to provide programs directed to employee relations.

Case 5.3 L'Hôpital St. Jean Baptiste Missionnaire

Dr. Michelle Ladot, from Lyons, France is a pediatrician at L'Hôpital St. Jean Baptiste Missionnaire in Akomey, Benin. The hospital is supported by La Société de Secours Étrangers in France. In addition to her regular clinic practice and emergency room duties, Dr. Ladot has been working with Dr. Emily Glass, a medical anthropologist from the United States, on a study of herbal medicines among the Pfau, a native people of central Benin.

The Pfau are one of the many African peoples that practice Sunna circumcision, a ritual known in the United States and Europe as *female genital mutilation (FGM)*. Despite government programs to curb the practice, some of which have been more successful since the 1994 International Conference on Population and Development in Cairo, the ritual persists. Current estimates are that over 2 million young women worldwide are subjected to the procedure annually. The prevalence of FGM among women aged 15–35 ranges from 72% in northern Ghana to 43% in Côte d'Ivoire and 20% in Senegal. Benin recently issued a public policy advisory against the practice.

Dr. Glass has been working closely with Abo Segu, one of the most respected herbalists in the region and a major religious leader. Abo Segu has been very concerned about infections leading to disabilities and even death from FGM. Although he supports the practice for religious reasons, he has tried to introduce less invasive procedures and sterile techniques.

After extensive and detailed discussions with Dr. Ladot, Dr. Glass and Abo Segu have proposed a new form of Sunna circumcision that would, according to Abo Segu, satisfy the traditional religious requirements. The new procedure involves only one minor incision and no removal of tissue. The young women would experience little or no pain, the chance of infection would be greatly reduced (even under less than sterile conditions), and sexual function (the ability to bear children) would remain normal. Because some nerves would be severed, however, sexual pleasure would be reduced in many women. Abo Segu and Dr. Glass propose that the new procedure be done by Dr. Ladot at L'Hôpital St. Jean Baptiste Missionnaire, with Abo Segu and others performing the religious ritual. If this works well, the procedure could be taught to the nurse clinicians who staff the field clinics. Eventually the whole practice might change—even when performed without medical supervision. Dr. Ladot is reluctant to perform medical procedures that have no health benefit but agrees to present the proposal to the hospital board.

Cases similar to this have been discussed at hospitals in the United States and Europe. The underlying problem of FGM is widespread (Dorkenoo, 1994). Conflicts between cultural norms can be almost irresolvable. How far should one go in compromising one's own principles in order to accommodate and respect the sincere practices of other people? Would this accommodation imply institutional approval of the ritual rather than a commitment to abolishing it? Given the fact that personal hygiene is no longer much of a health risk, would the practice really be much different than male circumcision, which presumably is already practiced in this Christian hospital?

CONCLUSIONS

Respect for individuals, regardless of race, religion, gender, disability, or other characteristics that have led to discrimination in the past, is an ideal that few people would question. Problem areas involve both conscious and unintentional personal attitudes that can conflict with optimal patient care. The elimination of sexual harassment and the accommodation of people with unconventional sexual orientations present challenges to develop organizational sensitivity to individuals. Development of institutional policies for effective affirmative action is a continuing and ever-changing responsibility. And the organizational response to intimate personal relationships in the workplace deserves careful management attention to individual rights.

Developing an organizational culture in which diversity is not only tolerated but valued, however, is not easy. Explicit principles included in organizational mission statements and professional and institutional codes of conduct can set the tone, but programs to develop and maintain these organizational commitments are needed as well. And there are, as some of the cases presented here demonstrate, conflicts of religious and cultural norms that can be very difficult to reconcile. The key here, it seems to me, is to identify and address these issues rather than to overlook or ignore them.

REFERENCES

ACHE (American College of Healthcare Executives), 1995, "Enhancing Minority Opportunities in Healthcare Management," http://www.ache.org/policy/policy5.html (2/7/99).

AIMD (American Institute for Managing Diversity), 1998, "Diversity Information Resource Center," http://www.aimd.org/ (3/4/98).

Anderson, Carol I., and Phillip L. Hunsaker, 1985, "Why There's Romancing at the Office and Why It's Everybody's Problem," *Personnel*, 62:57–63.

Anderson, Claire J., and Caroline Fisher, 1991, "Male–Female Relationships in the Workplace: Perceived Motivations in Office Romance," *Sex Roles*, 25(3–4):163–180.

BNA (Bureau of National Affairs), 1988, *Corporate Affairs: Nepotism, Office Romance, and Sexual Harassment*, Washington, DC, Bureau of National Affairs.

Boozang, Kathleen M., 1996, "Developing Public Policy for Sectarian Providers: Accommodating Religious Beliefs and Obtaining Access to Care," *Journal of Law, Medicine and Ethics*, 24:90–98.

Boyle, Philip J., and Mark J. Hanson, 1993, "Please Pass the Butter Cookies," *Hastings Center Report*, 23(3):28–29.

Capowski, Genevieve, 1996, "Managing Diversity," *Management Review*, 85(6):13–20.

Carnevale, Anthony Patrick, and Susan Carol Stone, 1995, *The American Mosaic*, New York: McGraw-Hill.

Colby, Lee, 1991, "Regulating Love," *Personnel*, 68(6):23.

Collins, Eliza G. C., 1983, "Managers and Lovers," *Harvard Business Review*, 61:140–152.

Dorkenoo, Efva, 1994, *Cutting the Rose: Female Genital Mutilation: The Practice and Its Prevention*, London: Minority Rights Publications.

DTG (Diversity Training Group), 1998, "Articles," www.diversitydtg.com/ (3/12/98).

Durkheim, Emile, 1906, "Détermination du fait moral," *Bulletin de la Société Française de Philosophie*, 6:113–139.

Fix, Michael, and Raymond J. Strucyk, eds., 1993, *Clear and Convincing Evidence: Measurement in America*, Washington, DC: Urban Institute Press.

Goldenring, John M., 1984, "Denial of Antipregnancy Prophylaxis to Rape Victims," *New England Journal of Medicine*, 311(25):1637.

HBS (Harvard Business School), 1991, "Ann Hopkins (A)" and "Ann Hopkins (B)," Boston, MA: Harvard Business School Publishing, www.hbsp.harvard.edu/bin/rotcgi (2/12/98).

Hopkins (*Hopkins v. Price Waterhouse*), 1985, 618 F Supp. 1109.

ICD (Institute for Corporate Diversity), 1996, *Diversity in Corporate America*, Minneapolis: Institute for Corporate Diversity.

Jamison, Kaleel, 1983, "Managing Sexual Attraction in the Workplace," *Personnel Administrator*, August, 45–50.

JCAHO (Joint Commission on Accreditation of Healthcare Organizations), 1996, *Comprehensive Accreditation Manual for Hospitals: The Official Handbook. Update, May, 1997*, Oakbrook Terrace, IL: Joint Commission on Accreditation of Healthcare Organizations.

Loden, Marilyn, 1996, *Implementing Diversity*, New York: Irwin.

Loewy, Erich H., 1994, "Institutional Morality, Authority, and Ethics Committees: How Far Should Respect for Institutional Morality Go?" *Cambridge Quarterly of Healthcare Ethics*, 3:578–584.

Mainiero, Lisa A., 1989, *Office Romance: Love, Power, and Sex in the Workplace*, New York: Rawson Associates.

MCHS (Multicultural Health Care Solutions), 1999, "Case Study," Bellaire, TX: Multicultural Health Care Solutions, http://www.mhcs.com/Default.htm (4/29/98).

Mead, Margaret, 1978, "A Proposal: We Need Taboos on Sex at Work," *Redbook*, April, 31–38.

NLGJA (National Lesbian and Gay Journalists Association), 1997, "Domestic Partner Benefits," www.nlgja.org/programs/DP/ (2/17/98).

OFCCP (Office of Federal Contract Compliance Programs), 1984, "OFCCP DIGEST: A Digest of Cases Under the Office of Federal Contract Compliance Programs," http://204.245.136.2/public/ofccp/refrnc/odigtc.htm (3/13/98).

Oncale (*Oncale v. Sundowner Offshore Services, Inc. et al.*), 1998, U.S. 96–568.

Orr, Robert D., 1995, "Should Religiously-Oriented Healthcare Institutions Have at Least One HEC Member with Opposing Views from the Institution's 'Standard Position'? No," *HEC Forum*, 7(6):367–369.

Post, Stephen G. and Leonard Fleck, 1995, "My Conscience, Your Money," *The Hastings Center Report*, 25(5):28–29.

Requena, 1986, "In the Matter of Beverly Requena," 213 N.J. Super 443.

SHRM (Society for Human Resource Management), 1991, *SHRM Privacy in the Workplace Survey Report*, Alexandria, VA: Society for Human Resource Management.

Siegel, Eugene, 1995, "Should Religiously-Oriented Healthcare Institutions Have at Least One HEC Member with Opposing Views from the Institution's 'Standard Position'? Yes," *HEC Forum*, 7(6):364–366.

St. Francis (St. Francis Health System, Pittsburgh, PA), 1999, "Philosophy," http://www.sfhs.edu/mission.html (3/15/99).

St. Joseph's Hospital (Ontario, Canada), 1998, "Our Values," http://www.stjosham.on.ca/mission.html (3/13/98).

Thomas, R. Roosevelt, Jr., 1991, *Beyond Race and Gender*, New York: AMACOM.

Velasquez, Manuel G., 1998, *Business Ethics: Concepts and Cases*, 4th ed., Upper Saddle River, NJ: Prentice-Hall.

Vinson (*Meritor Savings Bank v. Vinson*), 1986, 477 U.S. 57.

Wear, Stephen, 1991, "The Moral Significance of Institutional Integrity," *Journal of Medicine and Philosophy*, 16:225–230.

Williams, Robin M., 1959, *American Society: A Sociological Interpretation*, New York: Alfred A. Knopf.

6

PROGRAM DEVELOPMENT

Program development is not the sort of activity that can be captured in definite procedural steps. Even with the best planning, it is a free-flowing process that varies greatly with circumstances and among institutions. The ethical dimensions change accordingly: different situations raise different questions and require different solutions. The following discussion is presented not as a blueprint for program development, but as an example of the kinds of issues that can be expected to arise. Ethically, it employs the contextual approach, with more attention to the details of actual situations and relationships than to basic principles and values. Rather than providing a general account of the subject, the chapter employs a detailed case study. The case itself is something of a composite; it is based primarily on experience at a regional university hospital, but with two added features from another program.

Organizational change in health care is generally complex, but it is especially difficult in areas like organ procurement and transplantation services. Where various medical specialties are involved, there are clinical concerns regarding requests to the families of potential donors, and arrangements must be coordinated with an outside agency. The ethical issues raised by organ procurement and transplantation programs are diverse. The nature and timing of requests are matters of clinical ethics, the allocation of organs is a public policy matter, and there are several administrative issues involved in both. Program development in this area, furthermore, is now unavoidable: as of February 1999, all hospitals are required by federal regulations to have organ procurement programs. This chapter begins with some of the public policy issues, moves on to an example of program development, and then takes up aspects of organizational ethics. The final section raises some additional questions of distributive justice in the allocation of resources.

ORGAN TRANSPLANTATION

On February 26, 1998, Secretary of Health and Human Services Donna E. Shalala described the organ procurement situation in a letter to members of Congress in the following terms:

> We continue to have a serious shortage of organs for transplantation, and indeed in recent years, the shortage has grown worse. Some 55,000 persons are on the national organ transplant waiting lists today, up from 16,000 in 1988. More important, about 4,000 Americans died in 1996—almost 11 each day—while awaiting an organ transplant. It is estimated that we are achieving only about a third of our total potential for cadaveric organ donation. Improvement in bringing about organ donation would substantially reduce the number of Americans who die while awaiting a transplant, and that must be our first goal in improving our organ procurement and transplantation system.
>
> (Shalala, 1998)

While the number of donors did increase by 5.8% in 1998, the shortage is still serious; the number of African-American and Asian donors has not increased at all (UNOS, 1999). The technology is well developed and the success rate is improving, but sufficient organs are not available despite the fact that people say they are willing to donate. A 1993 Gallup poll showed that 69% of Americans would be likely to donate if asked (DHHS, 1998).

Under the National Organ Transplant Act of 1984, the United Network for Organ Sharing (UNOS), a not-for-profit organization, runs the Organ Procurement and Transplantation Network. The United Network for Organ Sharing is itself a federation of regional and local member organizations including every transplant program and regional organ procurement organization (OPO) for the recovery and allocation of organs in the United States. The policies of UNOS governing transplantation are developed through regional meetings and deliberations at the national committee level. Final approval is given by a 40-member board of directors composed of medical professionals, transplant recipients, and donor family members (UNOS, 1998a).

The United Network for Organ Sharing maintains the national Scientific Registry on Organ Transplantation to ensure that all patients have a fair chance of receiving organs, regardless of age, sex, race, lifestyle, religion, or financial or social status. Guidelines for allocation include physiological matching, medical urgency, consideration of local priorities, and time on the waiting list (UNOS, 1998b). Registry, allocation, and procurement are done primarily at the regional and local levels, where coordinators make the actual arrangements for donation. This process requires healthcare organizations that serve as donor and transplant centers to work cooperatively with the regional offices and coordinators.

Cooperative arrangements can be a source of friction. Physicians and surgeons may be reluctant to have organ procurement coordinators talk directly to patients' families. Organ procurement coordinators, however, are trained for this task and can often approach families with more experience and more sensitivity than physicians. In the midst of crucial medical situations where time for organ retrieval is of the essence, cooperative relationships are important but commonly difficult.

The shortfall in donations has prompted a number of actions. Some states have passed laws (following the model Uniform Anatomical Gift Act) that permit procurement of organs from anyone who dies with a valid organ donation card indicating his or her desire to be a donor. The organ donor card is legally sufficient, but OPOs have generally refrained from taking organs without consent of the next of kin since this would risk animosity that might turn public opinion against the program. The current National Organ and Tissue Donation Initiative of the Department of Health and Human Services has a goal of ensuring that all families are asked even if the donor has a signed consent form (HCFA, 1998). Another legal approach now in effect in many states is the *required request*, which mandates that families be approached concerning organ donation at the time of the death of a qualified donor. Required request laws have had little effect on improving donations because healthcare providers are reluctant to approach people in shock and sudden grief (DHHS, 1998).

One suggestion is to change the law so that it would be presumed that people will donate viable organs unless they specifically state otherwise, much as the law now contains a presumption to consent for resuscitation unless a medical order to the contrary has been written (Muyskens, 1978). Some states already have laws presuming consent for the removal of corneas for transplantation. The major objection to this proposal is based on the feeling that donation ought to be a free act rather than something that is required. Singapore has a dual system, with statutory donation and the ability to opt out for Singaporeans generally and no statutory requirement and the ability to opt in for Muslims (Rasheed, 1992).

Although direct monetary incentives such as the purchase of organs have been illegal in the United States since the passage of the National Transplantation Act in 1984, other incentives have been proposed. One proposal is that people who agree early in life to be donors should be given priority if they eventually need an organ. This might provide an incentive to some people, but it would be very difficult to administer. Another suggestion is that burial costs might be paid if a person agrees to be a donor; this would provide an incentive for survivor families (Jonson, 1997; McConnell, 1997:228–243). Since the current difficulty seems to be obtaining consent from the survivors, a donor card could also serve as a permission card. If the card includes a consent signed by the next of kin, the difficult step of requesting the donation might be facilitated (although it should probably not be eliminated). This would allow the donors themselves to obtain the necessary permission from their survivors to ensure that their wishes will be carried out.

The retrieval of organs is also a matter of continued debate in medical ethics. At present, organs are not often retrieved from people in a persistent vegetative state, from people on life support systems for an extended period of time, or from anencephalic infants. In these cases, obtaining organs often requires steps to be taken before death is declared, and the declaration of death is often not made on the basis of whole brain criteria. For example, courts have said that anencephalic infants are live human beings by existing criteria (the brain stem is functioning even though the upper brain may be absent) and, in some cases, must even be resuscitated and treated if the parents request it. In the case of people in persistent vegetative states from whom life support is withdrawn, the criterion of death is often cardiorespiratory failure rather than brain death and the organs become unusable due to lack of oxygenation. Suggestions have been made to use upper brain death as the criterion or to allow organ retrieval as life support is withdrawn, but this moves a step closer to taking organs while people are still alive. These considerations are clearly tied to a whole range of end-of-life problems, including physician assistance in dying, that have not been solved definitively in our society. In 1996 the AMA said that "physicians may provide anencephalic neonates with ventilator assistance and other medical therapies that are necessary to sustain organ perfusion and viability"—a step toward organ retrieval in these cases. But the AMA then added the condition that ventilator assistance should be maintained "until such time as a determination of death can be made in accordance with . . . law" (AMA, 1997:33). Organ procurement programs, perhaps wisely, have tended to keep out of this debate for fear that their motives will conflict with the interests of patients who are potential donors.

A Final Rule published by the Health Care Financing Administration (HCFA) in June 1998 requires more effective procurement measures (DHHS, 1998). Under this rule, all Medicaid and Medicare participating organizations must have agreements with a designated OPO to report all deaths. The OPO will determine the individual's suitability for donation and will cooperate with the hospital in the process of informing the family of the opportunity to donate organs. The Final Rule "ensures that only OPO representatives or trained individuals will approach families to explain their donation options and to make the actual request for donation" (DHHS, 1998:33856). The HCFA rule is based on current research.

> A retrospective review of all medically suitable potential donors referred to a single OPO in a one year period found a 67 percent consent rate when the OPO coordinator approached the family alone, a 9 percent consent rate when the hospital staff approached the family alone, and a 75 percent consent rate when the approach was made by the OPO coordinator and hospital staff together.
>
> (DHHS, 1998, 33856; referenced to Klieger et al., 1994)

This suggests that the current best practice is for a hospital-based health professional to first mention the donation option to the family and the OPO coordinator to make the request later. Studies cited in the HCFA's Final Rule also found a higher consent rate if the family was approached after notification of death so that they had time to come to grips with the situation.

The problem of finding enough organs for those in need is serious. Much will be lost if conflict between organ procurement programs and physicians or healthcare organizations exacerbates the problem. Good working relationships are essential, but healthcare organizations must also become more actively involved in education to increase the supply of organs. It is certainly appropriate for both healthcare administrators and clinical ethics committees to address this need, first to ensure that the best possible relationship between providers and the OPO is maintained and, second, to assist in both public and professional education.

Allocation of scarce resources has been an issue since the early days of medical ethics. It came to public attention when renal dialysis became available, but few dialysis machines were available and the cost was prohibitive. Congress responded by offering to pay for virtually all dialysis from the Social Security fund—the only health procedure for which the United States offers universal coverage. This answered the immediate need, but it raised many questions concerning the allocation of funds. Why should people with end-stage renal disease be offered universal coverage and not people with other medical conditions? Does the cost (about $1.2 billion annually) reduce what can be spent on other healthcare needs? And why should the money come from the Social Security fund?

While Congress was addressing the question of funding for this new lifesaving technology, the debate over who should receive dialysis was taking shape. At first, ethics committees were asked to make these decisions, but the idea of committees trying to decide among dialysis candidates based on their social merit (i.e., playing God) offended many people's feelings about equality (McConnell, 1997:216–218; Ramsey, 1970). While some commentators held that scarce resources ought to be allocated where they would do the most good, others argued that people should all have an equal opportunity, as in a lottery or waiting list procedure. The former position would require social criteria for deciding among candidates—a process human rights advocates generally reject. But the latter would permit some people who had recklessly injured themselves through high-risk behavior or unhealthy lifestyles to receive transplants. The idea of an unreformed alcoholic receiving a liver transplant is repugnant to many people.

This debate now seems to have been settled in favor of the random procedure, subject to initial medical matching and the practicalities of organ-sharing programs (UNOS, 1998b). Organ procurement programs continue to suffer serious consequences from publicity raising suspicions that a movie star or sports figure has been allowed to jump the queue. While celebrity is not considered once a person is on the waiting list, the inability to pay can keep a person off the list entirely (Caplan, 1999). In 1993 Governor Robert Casey of Pennsylvania received a heart-liver transplant one day after he was placed on the waiting list (McConnell, 1997:227).

Case 6.1 Program Development

Regional Medical Center (RMC), a 700-bed university-associated hospital in the Midwest, decided to develop a renal transplant program in 1992. Initial discussions at a transplant center in a neighboring state revealed that two transplant surgeons—one having just completed training and the other with extensive experience—would consider relocating to RMC for the purpose of starting their own program. A Certificate of Need application was developed with a successful study of the number of prospective patients in the service area. Three local nurses were sent for training at out-of-state transplant centers, and an experienced transplant nurse coordinator was recruited from another program. When the Certificate of Need was approved, orders were placed for the necessary equipment for a transplant surgical suite, and scheduling arrangements were made for availability of operating rooms on short notice. The major financial investment, as it turned out, was in the pathology department, which had to gear up for the different tests that would be needed. Hospital policies and procedures for procuring organs were reviewed for consistency with the new program. UNOS approved the new center for inclusion in its allocation program, and arrangements were made with the local OPO. Regional Medical Center had previously supplied organs to the local OPO, and the OPO was eager to have donated kidneys used locally. The nephrology group in the city was also happy to be able to refer patients for transplants locally and developed a cooperative relationship with the two renal transplant surgeons. Office space with clinic facilities for follow-up visits was arranged. When everything was in place, the first patients were admitted and, with appropriate public announcements, the transplant program was underway.

The program quickly established itself and in nine months was slightly ahead of the number of procedures projected. It had an excellent record. A year and a half into the program, however, signs of friction began to appear. The need for organs had grown faster than expected. Trauma surgeons had become aware of the need and felt pressure to obtain more donations. They had begun to discuss how far they should go in terms of keeping organs viable in patients who were alive but were not expected to survive. This raised questions that were brought to the clinical ethics committee: Should extra procedures be initiated for the sake of preserving organs for possible donation? What if these procedures actually prolonged the dying process?

Meanwhile OPO coordinators had become even more eager to talk to families of potential donors, and this had led to discussions of OPO procedures. Questions were raised about approaching the survivors of potential donors sooner after the death of a potential donor. The hospital policy for determining brain death required two flat electroencephalogram (EEG) readings six hours apart. One neurologist had suggested that if another reading was added four hours after the first, not to determine death but only for a status report to the family, it might be possible to begin the request process earlier. Whether allowing this additional time for the family to adjust would increase the number of donations was not known, however, and it was thought possible that an earlier approach would create the impression of a conflict of interest. The suggestion had also been made that trauma surgeons and critical care physicians be credentialed to declare death on the basis of brain criteria. This might facilitate the process of requesting donations in some cases.

Individual differences among the physicians had also begun to surface. Two neurologists and one trauma surgeon believed that physicians themselves rather than an OPO coordinator should discuss organ donation with the survivors. They felt that this was the most sensitive approach, since they would have been with the families through the tragic experience of the unexpected death. Two of these physicians had attended training programs for requestors; the third had not, and apparently believed that the attending physician should only mention the possibility of organ donation to the survivors rather than provide a longer explanation and make a more specific request. One neurologist, furthermore, had never really cooperated with the program. If the family had not mentioned organ donation before the patient's death, she assumed that they were not interested and disconnected support systems immediately after the second EEG reading and the declaration of brain death. She had, in fact, said that she considered it her duty to protect families from the OPO "agents." One reason for the suggestion of allowing trauma surgeons and critical care physicians to declare death on the basis of the second EEG was to bypass this uncooperative neurologist.

Other questions were raised by the nursing staff. As organ transplantation has become more common, families have begun to approach nurses with regard to possible donation. This often happens before the death of a patient. At first, the nurses were asked to refer the survivors to the OPO coordinator. This was not always practical, however, because some families wanted to discuss the matter before the patient's death and the OPO policy stated that this would be done only after death. Nurses continued to try to answer questions from families, and this inevitably led to more involved discussion. Furthermore, three nurses who were committed to the organ retrieval program had taken the training course for requesters, but this only made it less clear whether they should do this on a regular basis. Other nurses said that families asked about donating organs only if they were prepared to discuss the subject, and they believed that nurses should take advantage of the fact that the families had placed their trust in them.

All of this raised a number of questions: Should more emergency department and intensive care unit nurses be trained as requesters? How much time would be required for nurses to do this on a regular basis? Would this mean that the medical center was taking over some of the functions of the OPO or should these functions be clearly separated to avoid all appearance of a conflict of interest? Major administrators were also concerned. In two malpractice claims against the hospital, charges were made that families had been "harassed" by requests for organ donation. Two years into the operation of the RMC's organ transplantation program, then, there were a number of questions about professional roles and responsibilities, institutional policies and procedures, and cooperative agreements.

COMMENTS

Apart from the substantive matters involved in this case, there are important procedural issues. Some of the questions noted above concern organizational ethics, while others appear to be clinical ethics questions, medical staff matters, or managerial decisions. The question of when families should be approached regarding donation and the manner in which requests should be made would seem to be clinical ethics issues. The question of the roles and responsibilities of nurses and OPO coordinators, however, is an organizational matter. Dealing with reluctant or uncooperative physicians is both an organizational issue and a medical staff matter. The problems generated by the introduction of a new service unit as it interacts with existing services must be addressed at many levels within the organization.

Organizations facing difficult program coordination problems like these can begin to look for who is responsible. Ethics can be a matter of holding people responsible for what they have done wrong or what they could have done better. But while this may become necessary at times, finding individuals to blame isn't usually very helpful. As organizations grow or change, problems often develop. No one can foresee all the contingencies and consequences— especially when the consequences involve how people may react to organizational change. Prior to the opening of the transplant program, the people who were later upset may have thought there would be no problem. Ethical analysis can provide a way of identifying problems early by attempting to assess the various stakeholder interests and bringing the right people together to address the issues. It can also keep one's focus on the ultimate mission of the organization. Organizational ethics should be a way of solving problems, not a matter of finding out who is to blame when things go wrong.

This case demonstrates the extent to which ethical analysis is a normal dimension of organizational management. Organizational ethics questions are not separate from normal business management any more than bioethics questions are separate from medical issues. In this case, the ethical problems emerged after the full implications of the program became clear. Some people came to feel that better policies or procedures were needed; others felt pressured or were offended because they were expected to take on roles about which they had serious reservations; still others did not have a clear idea of what their role should be. Then in the normal friction of social life, some people became assertive and others became defensive. What procedures will be likely to work best and how functions can be coordinated has to be decided in light of the goals of the institution and the interests of all stakeholders.

In planning and program development, the major ethical issue is how an organization can remain faithful to its own mission and at the same time address the emerging needs of its many stakeholders. The first aspect is a matter of focus. Organizational mission statements seldom contain stated principles concerning planning and development, but organizations are institutions with past histories; they need to remain faithful to their historical tradition and to evaluate new opportunities and proposals in the light of their historical goals. The second aspect is a matter of confronting the needs of the people the organization serves in light of the capabilities of its professional staff and the resources it has available. There is a definite tension here; healthcare delivery has been a tumultuous field for the last quarter century. The fast pace of change, much of it driven by technical progress in medicine but some of it by a spirit of entrepreneurial venture, has led to some very poor planning. One hospital in a small eastern city became involved in an open heart surgery program because it wanted to keep up with medical progress, but also because two heart surgeons had moved to town and this presented what the hospital saw as a unique entrepreneurial opportunity. It was a bad move, especially since open heart surgery was offered by a program with a well-established reputation in a city less than 50 miles away. The program failed for lack of interest. Had the hospital kept more of a focus on its real mission, on the actual needs of the community, and on its own capabilities, it might have avoided the costly mistake.

Questions of planning and program development require both of the ethical perspectives presented here: the mission statement perspective to ensure focus and consistency with the tradition of the organization itself, and the stakeholder perspective to direct attention to the emerging needs of the external stakeholders and the actual capabilities of the internal stakeholders. Healthcare planning requires more than the identification of an unmet market demand. Studies can show a market even when a particular service would duplicate offerings being developed by other organizations in the area and even when the need identified is not the highest social priority. The fact that offering a new service can be successful financially is not an ethical mandate. From a utilitarian perspective, the course of action chosen must be the one that maximizes benefit considering the alternatives available. Healthcare program development should focus on the highest priority needs—which are not always those with the most immediate return on investment. Second, the ethical dimension of program planning requires attention to the people involved. Ethical analysis should include a process through which the interests of all people involved can be expressed and explored as plans are developed and before major friction occurs. Ethical analysis can play a preventive role.

These considerations raise a question that goes back to an issue of social responsibility discussed in Chapter 2. Should healthcare administrators be advocates for social causes or should they view their role as that of a neutral manager? The immediate answer to this question is that healthcare administrators should be more than bureaucratic managers and organizational ethics analysis should, indeed, be more than a compliance program. If ethical analysis is directed toward the fulfillment of the goals stated in an organizational mission statement, then the mission of the organization is the guiding light for social considerations. On the other hand, if the stakeholder approach is adopted, organizational ethics analysis would highlight stakeholder interests that might otherwise get neglected—especially the interests of the less powerful stakeholders. The socially concerned administrator is thus not required to bring some set of abstract values or personal beliefs into the organizational culture any more than other participants in the planning process are expected to do so. The task is more objective than this. The social values that the healthcare administrator should seek to advance are those that are intrinsic to the organization in the first place. Ethical analysis should serve as a "conscience" for the organization in the sense of calling on people to be mindful of the social goals to which the organization is already committed.

DISTRIBUTIVE JUSTICE

Finally, I turn to the question of distributive justice that is involved in many program development decisions. A number of years ago, the state health department in my state received an unexpected grant from the federal government to be used for primary care clinics. At that time the state had 29 clinics that offered services, mostly in rural areas, to patients on a sliding fee scale relative to household income. Some clinics were well established; others, in economically depressed areas, were struggling to make ends meet or to offer preschool vaccinations and prenatal care. There were also a few sections of the state that were not in any clinic service area at all. The larger cities, furthermore, had few clinic services since people tended to use hospital emergency rooms for primary care. In two cities, free clinics had just been established and had inquired about state support. When the federal grant became available, the state health department faced the question of allocation.

Legal counsel to the health department suggested that the funds should be divided according to the same percentage allocated to each clinic by the state legislature. The legislative allocation process, however, did not strike the administrators of the primary care program as necessarily the most rational. The legislature, they thought, simply gave more money to districts with powerful state senators and delegates. The state budget also reflected the historical fact that clinics that were first funded in prosperous times had received larger initial grants than those initially funded in more depressed years and that these funding levels tended to be carried over from year to year. No one was convinced that the legislative deliberation behind the state budget reflected much more than history and political power.

It was then proposed that the state program should establish a set of minimal standards (services offered) and that clinics should apply for funding from the federal grant on the basis of their track record. This procedure would allow the state program to set up a "basic minimum" guideline and to reward those clinics that were doing the best job. This was an incentive approach: clinics would find it in their interest to plan for and provide basic services so that they could compete effectively for funding.

A critic of this approach pointed out that the clinics already doing the best job would get the lion's share of the money and that these would be the clinics that were the best funded in the first place. They could even devote more resources to the grant application process. The only fair way to allocate the funds, this person said, would be to spread them evenly on a per-capita basis. The funds should be divided according to the population of each service area.

A final proposal was based on the recognition that distribution of resources on a per-capita basis would not address the problems of those who were most in need. Some sections of the state, in fact, were wealthier than others, and there was less need (per-capita) in those areas. From this perspective, an indicator of actual need, such as the unemployment rate or the percentage of families receiving income support, should be used for the allocation. The decision should also take into account the problems of the free clinics that were responding to severe needs with no state support and other areas of the state that had no clinic coverage.

There are various criteria of distributive justice that can be applied to this problem with some sense of fairness. The mission of the state agency, however, is to bring primary care to as many people as possible, so the proposal based on need would arguably be the most appropriate. There is also a question of governmental ethics involved here. Should appointed state officials rely only on legislative determinations (i.e., follow the state budget) or should they exercise independent judgment based on the established goals by making their own determination of social needs (Henry, 1975)?

Case 6.2 The Oregon Medicaid Program
The question of distributive justice is also illustrated by the Oregon Health Plan. Beginning in 1989, the state of Oregon made a number of changes in its health care system. Collectively, the intent of the reforms was to expand insurance coverage to all state residents. Many provisions of the plan were politically progressive and had been discussed in other states. The establishment of a high-risk health insurance pool for people who had been refused coverage was similar to the automobile insurance pool programs in many states. As of 1996 the high-risk pool insured 4300 residents. A second state program made health insurance available to over 27,000 people working in small businesses. A third initiative mandating that employers either provide health insurance or pay into a state fund required federal enabling legislation that was never passed, so this never took effect.

The most noteworthy component of the Oregon plan was the move to expand Medicaid coverage to all state residents with incomes below the federal poverty level. It was projected that as many as 180,000 additional state residents would qualify for Medicaid. To finance this expansion of the Medicaid program, the state initiated two cost-containment mechanisms. The first requires Medicaid patients to join a managed care program. The second is a prioritized list of services that is theoretically the most interesting aspect of the Oregon Health Plan.

The priority list is, in fact, a means of rationing health care by simply excluding from Medicaid coverage services that have a low priority. Oregon established a Health Services Commission that, through a series of opinion surveys, community meetings, and Commission deliberations, drew up a list of health services ranging from high to low priority. Since the demand for each service could be predicted from past experience and the average cost of each service could be calculated, the Oregon Health Plan could determine what it would cost the state to fund services on the priority list above any given point. Alternatively, if the legislature set the funding for Medicaid at a certain level, Plan administrators could tell which services that level of funding would exclude. In 1994 and 1995, for example, the Plan covered the first 606 of the 745 items on the list.

By some quantitative measures, the Oregon Health Plan has been successful. Emergency room visits were down by 4%–5%—more in rural areas than in urban areas. In 1994 charity care declined by 18.7% and bad debts by 10.6%. Both continued to fall through 1995—more in urban areas than in rural areas. Changes in the Medicaid part of the Plan since 1995 have included the addition of mental health services through managed care contracts and a rise in the threshold from line 606 on the priority list to line 581. Services at the low-priority end of the list tend to be less effective, as well as being judged less essential (Conviser, 1998).

The rationing of services under the Oregon Health Plan has been criticized in a number of ways. The most significant objection is that it expands the number of Medicaid recipients by taking away benefits from people who had previously been receiving them (Daniels, 1991). If the priority list actually allocates funds to more beneficial services, however, its use would increase both the number of people covered and the total amount of benefit. The criteria here are the public goals of the Plan and fair treatment of those who have a stake in it.

CONCLUSIONS

Planning and program development, whether in individual healthcare organizations or at the level of public policy, involve many problems. Some are clinical issues, others are operational matters, and still others are policy questions. Ethical guidance in solving these problems can be derived from the analytical perspectives employed here. Administrators and other professionals involved in the planning process need to keep in mind the mission of the organization and the many people who will be affected by organizational change.

It may seem simplistic to say that program planning ought to be guided by the ultimate goals of the organization and ought to take account of the interests of those who will be affected by it. But these ethical aspects of planning decisions often get lost in the evaluation of alternatives, the effort to comply with regulations, or the consideration of pressure from powerful interests. The ethical mandate may be simple, but its implementation can be complex. It is all too easy for administrators and practitioners concerned about the success of their own divisions to lose sight of the organization's goals and the many people who will be affected by their decisions and actions.

REFERENCES

AMA (American Medical Association), 1997, *Code of Medical Ethics: Current Opinions with Annotations*, Chicago: American Medical Association.

Caplan, Arthur, 1999, "With Transplants, Celebrity can Help," http://www.med.upenn.edu/bioethics/breaking/3Feb99.html (5/14/99).

Conviser, Richard, 1998, "A Brief History of the Oregon Health Plan and Its Features," http://www.ohppr.state.or.us/ (4/29/98).

Daniels, Norman, 1991, "Is the Oregon Rationing Plan Fair?" *Journal of the American Medical Association*, 265(17):2232–2235.

DHHS (Department of Health and Human Services), 1998, "Health Care Financing Administration Final Rule," *Federal Register*, June 28, 63(119):33856.

HCFA (Health Care Finance Administration Press Office), 1998, "National Organ and Tissue Donation Initiative," http://waisgate.hhs.gov/cgi-bin/waisgate?WAISdocID = 365513215 + 0 + 0 + 0&WAISaction = retrieve (5/17/99).

Henry, Nicholas, 1975, *Public Administration and Public Affairs*, Englewood Cliffs, NJ: Prentice-Hall.

Jonsen, Albert R., 1997, "Ethical Issues in Organ Transplantation," in Robert. M. Veatch, ed., *Medical Ethics*, 2nd ed., Boston: Jones and Bartlett Publishers.

Klieger, J., Nelson K., Davis R., et al., 1994, "Analysis of Factors Influencing Organ Donation Consent Rates," *Journal of Transplant Coordination*, 4:132.

McConnell, Terrance, 1997, *Moral Issues in Health Care: An Introduction to Medical Ethics*, 2nd ed., Belmont, CA: Wadsworth Publishing Company.

Muyskens, James L., 1978, "An Alternative Policy for Obtaining Cadaver Organs for Transplantation," *Philosophy and Public Affairs*, 8:88–99.

Ramsey, Paul, 1970, *The Patient as Person*, New Haven, CT: Yale University Press.

Rasheed, H.Z.A., 1992, "Organ Donation and Transplantation—A Muslim View," *Transplantation Proceedings*, 24(5):2116–2117.

Shalala, Donna, 1998, "Letter to Members of Congress," February, 26, http://www.unos.org/frame_Default.asp?Category = About (3/17/98).

UNOS (United Network for Organ Sharing), 1998a, "Who We Are," http://www.unos.org/frame_Default.asp?Category = About (3/17/98).

——, 1998b, "Policies," http://www.unos.org/frame_Default.asp?Category = About (3/17/98).

——, 1999, "Cadaveric Organ Donation Increased 5.6 Percent in 1998," http://www.unos.org/frame_Default.asp?Category = Newsroom (5/14/99).

7

MEDICAL RECORDS

> What I may see or hear in the course of the treatment, or even
> outside of the treatment in regard to the life of men, which on no
> account one must spread abroad, I will keep to myself holding
> such things shameful to be spoken about.
>
> Hippocrates (Arras and Steinbock, 1995:54)

The confidentiality of medical and personal information is a principle as old as
Hippocrates and as modern as the most recent version of the AMA Code of
Ethics:

> The information disclosed to a physician during the course of the relationship be-
> tween physician and patient is confidential to the greatest possible degree.
>
> (AMA, 1997:77)

The new version of the principle is, in certain respects, just as out of date as
the old one. Both appear to presume that medical care is a matter of one physician in a relationship with one patient, with the information limited to what the
patient discloses. Today, with multiple physicians, other specialists, laboratory
technicians, nurses, clerks, medical students, social workers, chaplains, researchers, medical committees, administrative committees, quality review auditors, admitting clerks, billing clerks, and a whole corps of approval officers,
financial intermediaries, and insurance processors all involved, medical information seems to be anything but confidential. The problem is further exacerbated by the variety of ways in which information can be stored and transferred
electronically, and by the ease with which paper or electronic copies can be
made (Thompson, 1992). As Mark Siegler wrote in 1982 with only a certain

amount of overstatement, "Medical confidentiality as it has traditionally been understood by patients and doctors, no longer exists" (Siegler, 1999:169)

This gradual erosion of personal privacy is to a large extent a result of medical progress. Medical care now requires a team approach, so more medical professionals need to know about the patient. Expansion of the medical model to include psychological, social, and economic issues has widened the circle of disclosure even further. With these developments in the nature of medical care, the problem of confidentiality itself has changed. The question of when and why physicians should disclose information given to them in confidence is still important, but it is being eclipsed by questions about the security of this information in medical records systems. Confidentiality is now an organizational problem.

SECURITY, ACCESS, AND CONSENT

With respect to the privacy of personal information, an important distinction should be made between the security of information and access to it. *Security* refers to whether an unauthorized person can obtain information. Electronic storage of medical records and transmission of data by fax or via the Internet create the danger of unauthorized individuals or companies obtaining confidential information. Although this problem has received considerable attention in the media and involves a number of technical issues, it does not raise especially difficult ethical questions since few people would want to defend anyone who obtains medical records illegally.

Legal access is the more serious problem from an ethical perspective. While public attention has been diverted to the issue of security of medical records from unauthorized use, the circle of authorized access has been expanding. Medical information legally disclosed to employers, for example, may be used (legally or illegally, depending on the state) for employment decisions. "In 1995," according to Joanne Silberner, "University of Illinois researchers surveyed Fortune 500 Companies and found that 35 percent said they used medical information to make decisions about hiring and firing" (Silberner, 1997:8). According to a recent report by the JCAHO and the NCQA, "the most common abuses stem from misuse of personal health information by legitimate users with authorized access to personal health records" (JCAHO/NCQA, 1998).

The "Prologue" to the JCAHO/NCQA report "Protecting Personal Health Information: A Framework for Meeting the Challenges in a Managed Care Environment" contains the following examples:

> A health plan conducts a quality review that highlights issues in the management of the care of their diabetic patients. To improve quality of care, the health plan contracts with a disease management company to oversee their diabetic patients. As

part of this contract, the health plan supplies a computerized record of their members with a diagnosis of diabetes. Without any prior notice, the health plan's members begin to receive calls from the disease management firm to discuss their diabetic care. A number of members are alarmed to find that their personal health information has been shared with a party of which they have no knowledge.

A pharmacy benefits management (PBM) company is acquired by a pharmaceutical manufacturer. The pharmaceutical company has begun to market a new drug for the treatment of asthma. This medication has been shown to be significantly more effective than other drugs on the market. The pharmaceutical company decides to mount a campaign to inform patients about this new medication. One of their strategies is to identify individuals under its PBM who have had prescriptions filled for other asthma medications. An information packet on the new medication is mailed to each of these patients.

(JCAHO/NCQA, 1998)

Federal law offers little or no protection against authorized access to medical information. Information released to one insurance company for reimbursement purposes may be passed on to other companies and used to deny or limit insurance coverage. The Medical Information Bureau (MIB) is a Massachusetts-based insurance reporting agency that holds medical records on about 15 million Americans and Canadians and distributes reports to over 750 insurance firms. In the absence of legislation regulating medical information, however, the procedures and practices of MIB could be addressed only through consumer laws. In 1995 the FTC forced MIB to abide by federal regulations that protect consumers from unfair treatment in credit checks (FTCBCP, 1995).

Under the new rule, . . . all insurance companies who [sic] are members of the MIB will abide by the Fair Credit Reporting Act requirement that an individual be informed when a consumer report [i.e., the medical report from MIB] played any part in the insurer's decision to deny coverage or to charge a higher rate. In such cases, the insurance company will notify the consumer of the name and address of the consumer reporting agency [i.e., MIB] that provided the report. Consumers who receive the notice are entitled to receive a free copy of their report from the reporting agency, if requested within 30 days, to verify that all information is correct.

(FTCBCP, 1995)

The amount of private information held and made available might surprise many people. "In addition to an individual's credit history, data collected by MIB may include medical conditions, driving records, criminal activity, and participation in hazardous sports, among other facts" (FTCBCP, 1995). The MIB information is held and used, according to the Office of Technology Assessment, "solely for the purpose of assisting the insurance industry in making coverage exclusions" (OTA, 1993:30). It has also been reported that insurance companies are now asking physicians to collect information on patients that would more properly be characterized as lifestyle information rather than health records (Breitenstein, 1997). The distribution of medical records and other information by MIB is all done legally, of course. Patients have signed general consent forms or blanket waivers to permit their insurance companies to see their medical records, and there is no violation of privacy if the insurance company uses this information for its own business purposes.

The critical issue with regard to legal access to health records is the question of consent. Patients do, of course, sign consent forms for the release of medical records, but their consent is seldom fully informed and can hardly be characterized as voluntary. It is not informed because patients are not notified of the people who will have access to their information or the purposes for which it will be used. Once a consent form is signed, disclosure is entirely up to the organization to which permission for disclosure has been given. And it should not go unnoticed here that consent is given to an organization, not to an individual. The patient cannot, in fact, be fully informed of the extent of disclosure of his or her information at the time of consent because the organization may later decide to release it for some other use. Healthcare organizations generally retain the right to decide on their own whether release of patient records is warranted.

The most crucial aspect of the problem of consent is perhaps the most obvious: consent to disclosure of information is not voluntary. Unless consent is given, payment for services will not be authorized. Faced with pressing healthcare needs, and with hospitals and insurance plans that require permission to disclose records, the patient has little choice. According to the Office of Technology Assessment, "since individuals are, for the most part, not able to forego health care reimbursement benefits, they really cannot make a meaningful choice whether or not to consent to disclosure of their health care information" (OTA, 1993:17). With the expansion of health services beyond the individual doctor–patient relationship, voluntary informed consent for the disclosure of confidential information has been replaced by coerced, uninformed consent.

ETHICAL PERSPECTIVES

Confidentiality is considered important for two reasons. First, the disclosure of certain personal information is essential to diagnosis and treatment, and patients will be willing to share private information only if they believe that it will be kept confidential. A second reason relates to the notion of personal integrity or dignity. Each of us has a private dimension to our life—a realm of uncertain, even tentative thoughts, feelings, fears, and emotions. This private realm is essential to the growth and development of the public persona we present to others. It can be important to reveal parts of our private selves to our closest friends whose good will we trust—and to physicians who may need to know about private matters in order to treat us. But we also protect the privacy of this inner personal life so that we have room to change as we grow and develop without being so public that we get tagged with labels we may not want later. When private aspects of our lives are exposed to the public around us, we lose some freedom to manage our self-presentation. The private dimension of our lives is important to us personally, and preserving it is an essential part of personal integrity or dignity.

Organizational mission statements seldom mention the confidentiality of medical information. In the past, this was not necessary. In Western culture, confidentiality of medical information has been presumed to be a matter of professional ethics. One would expect to find the principle of confidentiality in the AMA Code of Ethics and in similar codes of other healthcare professionals, not necessarily in an organizational mission statement. The AMA Code is, in fact, more explicit than the single statement quoted above. It goes on to say:

> The patient should feel free to make a full disclosure of information to the physician in order that the physician may most effectively provide needed services. The patient should be able to make this disclosure with the knowledge that the physician will respect the confidential nature of the communication. The physician should not reveal confidential communications or information without the express consent of the patient, unless required to do so by law.
>
> (AMA, 1997:77)

There is a body of opinion in two sections of the AMA Code that builds on these principles and covers many specific situations, such as care for minors, attorney–physician relations, disclosure to insurance companies, and transfer of information between physicians.

If it could be presumed that what a physician writes in a hospital medical record is kept within a circle of strict confidentiality by a healthcare organization, a physician might still claim that he or she was not revealing confidential information without the patient's express consent. But now, with the expanding distribution of medical records and the blanket nature of consent forms, the AMA Code makes little sense. In fact, the only thing that keeps it from being outright deceitful is that it uses the term "express consent" rather than "voluntary informed consent." Patients do give express consent, but they are uninformed and, at least indirectly, coerced. Since medical records are now held and used by healthcare organizations as well as by individual physicians, the confidentiality of medical information is no longer just a professional matter.

On the organizational level, principles regarding confidentiality are often required by accreditation standards and are generally found in various statements of patient's rights. Perhaps the most widely used patient's bill of rights is the one published by the AHA. It addresses confidentiality in forceful terms:

> The patient has the right to expect that all communications and records pertaining to his/her care will be treated as confidential by the hospital, except in cases such as suspected abuse and public health hazards when reporting is permitted or required by law.
>
> (AHA, 1992)

The AHA patient's bill of rights also states that "the patient has the right to expect that the hospital will emphasize the confidentiality of this information when it releases it to any other parties entitled to review information in these records." Unfortunately, it says only that the hospital must "emphasize" confidentiality, not that the hospital must assure it with appropriate requirements. The bill also leaves it up to the hospital to decide, on its own, which parties are entitled to review records. It does not require patient consent for research or commercial use; nor does it require that patients be informed when their records are released.

The actual practice of healthcare organizations with regard to disclosure and consent is little better than current legal protection. Hospitals tend to use blanket consent forms and decide later who will be allowed access to records and for what purposes. A recent study showed that only 41% of university-affiliated hospital consent forms identified the organization as a teaching institution and gave notice that medical and other professional students would have access to records (Merz et al., 1998). Only 19% specifically disclosed the use of records for medical research, and only 45% disclosed release for quality review purposes. While release of information for insurance purposes was almost universally obtained, the authors did not report whether medical records could be passed along to other insurance companies or to employers. As things stand now, therefore, institutional policies are not much stronger than federal and state regulations. Attempts by individual physicians to address the problem, furthermore, can lead to difficulties. Consider the following case.

Case 7.1 Personal Notes

Dr. Susan Miller, a psychiatrist, has become concerned about the freedom with which hospital staff members talk about patient information that she considers confidential. A certain amount of discussion is unavoidable, but this should be limited, she thinks, to what is necessary for professional care. Thus, she has begun to keep her own private notes on her patients. She puts what she considers necessary in the chart but notes anything else she wants to remember in a small notebook she carries. This is often information about a patient's family or particular points about a patient's history. Her patients know that she keeps her own information separate from hospital records, and some have said that they appreciate her concern for confidentiality.

The hospital staff, however, doesn't appreciate this. On occasions when Dr. Miller's patients have been seen by resident physicians, the residents have felt that important aspects of the patients' conditions may have been omitted from the record. In some cases, it was not entirely evident why Dr. Miller had prescribed certain medications; in other cases, support staff members felt that they should have had a better understanding of patients. It was not clear, however, whether the medical record might have contained more information or whether the staff just felt that Dr. Miller was being secretive. Eventually the nurse manager of the Behavioral Medicine Department raised the question with the medical director: should a physician be keeping private case notes on patients apart from the medical record?

In this case, Dr. Miller appears to be concerned both with the confidentiality of medical records themselves and with the organizational culture in which patients' stories are shared too freely. Both issues need to be addressed: how to keep the records held more closely and how to keep the staff from gossiping. Then there is the question of the propriety of Dr. Miller's practice of keeping "double books." There may be legal aspects to this practice if the official records are incomplete, as well as managerial and clinical dimensions involving staff relations and responsibilities.

PROPOSED SOLUTIONS

The 1974 Privacy Act (PL 93–579) established certain conditions and procedures for handling medical records, set definite limits on disclosure of information that can be linked to individuals, and even provided civil and criminal penalties for violations. This law applies only to federal agencies, however. The 1996 Kennedy-Kassebaum bill (PL 104–191) established a 1999 deadline for further Congressional action; if Congress didn't meet the deadline, the Department of Health and Human Services was authorized to establish its own guidelines. Congress did not act and the Department has now published guidelines that require:

a. that patients be able to obtain copies of their medical records,
b. that patients be permitted to request changes if they believe their medical records contain errors,
c. that providers be required to indicate how they will store and handle medical information,
d. that patients be allowed to designate who will have access to records, with specific consent for disclosure other than for treatment and payment purposes,
e. that civil and criminal penalties be imposed for security violations,
f. that administrative subpoena will be required for disclosure to law enforcement agents, and
g. that federal regulations would not pre-empt stricter state laws.

(DHHS, 1999)

Hospitals, insurers, pharmaceutical companies, and health plans objected in advance to the provision requiring patient approval for disclosure. Hospitals do not want to deal with permission forms every time they disclose information for a new purpose. Insurers and health plans want to be able to use records for cost control, and pharmaceutical companies want to continue to use patient data for research and marketing purposes. In November 1998 the JCAHO and the NCQA warned that forceful access regulations may have a negative impact on patient care, medical research, public health programs, and even consumer information (Pretzer, 1999).

On the other side of the debate, civil rights organizations have objected to the fact that the administrative rules give free access to medical information to law enforcement agencies on the basis of administrative subpoena. A. G. Breitenstein of the JRI Health Law Institute has stated that physicians may have to warn patients that anything they say may be used against them in a court of law (Breitenstein, 1997). Legislation introduced by Senator Robert F. Bennett would require law enforcement officials to obtain a search warrant or a subpoena from a court (Carey, 1997).

The new federal rules are of limited effect, however, since they only apply to providers and insurers, and leave pharmaceutical companies, employers, and other organizations to whom medical information is passed entirely unregulated. The situation is still fluid: Congress could act at any time to override the Department's rules. And regardless of what legal requirements are mandated at federal or state levels, healthcare organizations will still have to consider their own policies. At this time, therefore, the major issue before the country is still whether patients' medical records will be legally available only for treatment and payment purposes, or whether they will remain available to life insurers, employers, pharmaceutical companies, and health plans for a wide range of business purposes (Givens, 1997; HLI, 1996; OTA, 1993). Even journalists are demanding greater access (Campbell, 1998).

Rather than attempt to predict what may happen during the next few years, I will offer a brief list of ethical principles that are relevant both to legislation and to the implementation of organizational policies and procedures. In formulating this list, I draw first on the basic principles of fair information practice described in a report published by the Department of Health, Education and Welfare in 1973 (in OTA, 1993).

1. *There must be no secret personal data system; there must be a way for individuals to discover what information is kept on them.* It is hoped that the debate about patients' access to their own medical records is just about over. Except in cases of incompetence and medical indications to the contrary, there is little reason for keeping medical records from patients themselves. Informed consent requires knowledge. There can be no informed consent to the release of data if one doesn't know what the record contains.

2. *There must be a way for individuals to prevent information about them obtained for one purpose from being used or made available for other purposes.* Whether this is best done through controlling access by requiring consent for each new use or through explicit and enforceable use restrictions must still be worked out. Under the Americans with Disabilities Act, for example, there is a use restriction. Employers can hold medical records of employees in a secured way, but they are not permitted to use those records for employment decisions other than in areas related to a disability accommodation. Requiring separate consent for commercial use (defined as any use that is of commercial value outside of the context of treatment), certain types of insurance use, and any research use in which patients are identifiable may be an alternative to requiring permission each time. People do need assurance that confidential information about themselves will not be used for purposes other than those agreed to or established in law; but if the scope of legal use is limited, this will provide some assurance.

3. *An organization maintaining or disseminating records of identifiable personal data must ensure the reliability of the data for their intended use, and there must be a way for individuals to correct or amend their medical records.* If medical records are to be used in as many ways as now seems likely, patients must have the ability to make sure that the records are accurate. This implies a responsibility on the part of healthcare organizations to be reasonably certain of the accuracy of medical information, and to release it only with assurances that the next holder will use it solely for the purposes indicated and will not pass it along without similar restrictions.

4. *Consent for disclosure must be voluntary and informed.* Given the complexity of the matter, methods will have to be found to guarantee that patients understand the nature of the information they are asked to release and its intended use. Whether coercion can be entirely eliminated is doubtful, but the use restrictions mentioned above would certainly make consent easier for many patients if medical use were clearly separated from commercial use.

5. *Access to medical records by law enforcement officials and civil litigants should be limited by due process protections.* While no one can search your house without a warrant or compel you to produce tax records or other papers without a subpoena, the same is not true of medical records held by healthcare providers. Although many healthcare organizations do not now grant access to medical records unless they are legally required to do so, search warrants should be mandatory (Perrone, 1997).

6. *The flow of medical information should be documented.* Improper disclosure of medical information cannot be detected without a record. There is no reason to allow access to information without noting the disclosure in the information itself. Physicians and hospitals now generally track access to medical records, but tracking should be required by law. With the electronic storage and networking of information, tracking of authorization (who approved disclosure) and access (who received the record) should pose no great problems.

7. *Security measures for electronic data processing should be mandatory.* The fast pace of technological developments makes it impossible to specify exactly what will be necessary to maintain the security of medical information in the future. The following guidelines, proposed in 1993 by Vincent M. Brannigan, will give some idea of what might be needed (OTA, 1993:86; see also Krause and Brown, 1996). According to Brannigan, electronic data systems should

1. control authorized requesters by use of restricted request software needed to access the database;
2. protect passwords used to identify individual requesters;
3. route requests through a secure electronic mail system that eliminates direct electronic connection to the data bank;
4. allow searches only by patient name, and prevent random browsing of the databank;
5. provide an audit trail to the individual subject;
6. maintain a secure data facility not connected to the health institution;
7. allow responses to be sent in a secure manner, only to pre-approved addresses;
8. provide the individual subject a way to monitor disputed, incorrect, or un-needed data;
9. require encryption and transmission through secure electronic mail to a mail-box accessible only to users with authorized decryption software;
10. permit searches only for authorized purposes;
11. allow searches only with the permission of that patient.

(OTA, 1993)

Confidentiality will continue to pose serious problems for organizations, but the enactment of provisions based on principles such as these will go a long way toward protecting patients (Nagel, 1997; Privacy Rights Clearinghouse, 1997).

THE PUBLIC VALUE OF MEDICAL INFORMATION

Privacy is not the only value involved in the issue of medical information, however. Lawrence O. Gostin, former chair of the Privacy Working Group of the President's Task Force on National Health Care Reform, has argued that the right to confidentiality is neither absolute nor intrinsic and that it must be balanced against the public good. Health information can be used to promote access to health care, more equitable distribution of services to vulnerable populations, better research, and more effective public health interventions. These uses, according to Gostin, are ethically appropriate (Gostin, 1995). The purpose of government, he points out, is to achieve collective goals that individuals acting alone could not achieve, and health promotion, as one of these goals, requires the collection and use of health information.

Individuals already forego significant levels of privacy in order to obtain the social goods that benefit society collectively. Many of the collective goals in society, ranging from law enforcement and public safety to tax collection and national security, are achieved partly by substantial collection of personal information. . . . As the United States intensely considers the value and effectiveness of its health care system, it must acknowledge that one of the burdens of achieving cost effective and accessible care is a loss of privacy.

(Gostin, 1995:515)

Gostin's point is well taken: insistence on absolute privacy for health information will inhibit the attainment of other health benefits. This implies that we should seek a balance that will protect individual privacy while permitting beneficial use of medical records. This is not, however, what we currently have. I believe that people would generally permit the use of their medical records for research or public health purposes if they had confidence in the security of the system and the elimination of unwarranted commercial access. Gostin himself would require removal of patient identification from research data or the use of coding if identification is necessary. He also argues for specific use limits, independent review of the value of research, and fully informed consent. The use of medical information for public health purposes, therefore, would not be inconsistent with the procedures listed above.

Finally, there is a problem that will never be solved by legal regulations or institutional policies. This is the situation in which information is inadvertently disclosed. Consider the following case.

Case 7.2 Illegal Information

The Administrative Director of Patterson Memorial Hospital, Cheryl Truman, received a call from John Scott, Director of Human Resources. Patterson Memorial is a 180-bed community hospital, one of two community hospitals in a small industrial city in the South. Mr. Scott said that he needed some advice on a problem brought to him by Dr. George Sawyer, who assists with the hospital benefits program. The program routinely offers health screenings, flu shots, and other services free to hospital employees. Last week an operating room nurse, Susan White, came in with a request for a blood test for a marriage license. She brought her fiancee along for his test as well. The laboratory report came back to Dr. Sawyer, who was supposed to sign the form.

"The problem," Mr. Scott explained, "is that the lab report says Susan tested HIV positive." "Of course," he said, "the lab wasn't supposed to run an HIV test at all; you can't do that in this state without explicit written permission—it's illegal. I called the pathologist, and he apologized; he said I should just throw that part of the report out. The test was run with two other blood tests that day, and the technician apparently thought they were all the same. I'm not sure about just throwing it out; I asked Dr. Sawyer about Susan's fiancee. His blood tested HIV negative. Of course, we weren't supposed to know that either. We got the information by mistake, but Dr. Sawyer thinks he should tell Susan and her fiancee." Ms. Truman said she would think about it and call back.

The next day Mr. Scott called Ms. Truman again. "Dr. Sawyer decided he had an obligation to tell Susan," he said. "She was furious. She didn't know she was HIV positive. She said she was in New York for about two years, and when her marriage broke up, she was living in the fast lane for a while before she moved back here. But that was five years ago. Then, two hours later, she called Dr. Sawyer again and told him that she had decided not to tell her fiancee and said he could not tell her fiancee either. She said this was her medical information, and no one else had a right to it. In fact, she was worried about the pathologist and the lab technician. So am I: you know how things are around here. I'm not even sure I should have told you! I don't know if this should affect her employment. Sawyer says he is worried about an HIV-positive nurse working in surgery; that's asking for trouble. What if this got to the newspaper? Sawyer also thinks he has to tell her fiancee, but he said he would wait until I talk with you."

While the information here was generated by mistake and passed along without much consideration, this situation is not unusual. Still, people and organizations have to take responsibility for their mistakes. The Director of Human Resources and the Administrative Director were informed in the course of an attempt to deal with the problem. Did Dr. Sawyer complicate the problem by disclosing it to the Human Resource Director? Was it complicated further when Cheryl Truman was informed? Could the issue have been handled without disclosing the identities of the parties involved? In most states, the law permits a state health officer to disclose or to authorize a physician to disclose the risk of a sexually transmitted disease to a sexual contact. It can be as difficult to control the informal spread of information as to keep medical records secure.

CONCLUSIONS

Medical confidentiality is an organizational problem. As the expansion of medical care into a team approach has widened the circle of those who have a need to know, the focus has shifted from security of medical information to the issue of access. Technology, bureaucracy, and medical specialization have seriously eroded the once private doctor–patient relationship. Current safeguards are inadequate: insurance companies can disclose confidential information for business purposes, and healthcare organizations use blanket disclosure forms that allow extended access. We need newer and stronger regulations to limit authorized access to information. At present, organizations can remind employees and associated professionals of the importance of confidentiality, but this does not address the organizational nature of the issue. Healthcare organizations need to review the flow of information within their systems in light of their own commitments to their patients. Promises made to patients in organizational mission statements and the patient's bill of rights must be backed up by explicit provisions in organizational codes of conduct making it clear that unauthorized disclosure of information is a serious offense.

REFERENCES

AHA (American Hospital Association), 1992, "A Patient's Bill of Rights," http://www. aha.org/resource/pbillofrights.html (12/4/99).

AMA (American Medical Association), 1997, *Code of Medical Ethics: Current Opinions and Annotations*, 1996–1997 edition, Chicago: American Medical Association.

Arras, John D., and Bonnie Steinbock, 1995, *Ethical Issues in Modern Medicine*, 4th ed., Mountain View, CA: Mayfield Publishing Company.

Breitenstein, A. G., 1997, "Testimony (to the Senate Committee on Labor and Human Resources)," October 28, 1997, http://www.jrihealth.org/programs/law/privrec.shtml (4/22/98).

Campbell, Joel, 1998, "Congress, States Plan Assault on Access to Medical Records," *Quill*, 86(1):38.

Carey, Mary Agnes, 1997, "Privacy of Medical Records Under Hill Microscope," *Congressional Quarterly Weekly Report*, 55(43):2682–2689.

DHHS (U.S. Department of Health and Human Services), 1999, "Proposed Standards for Privacy of Individually Identifiable Health Information," http://aspe.os.dhhs.gov/admnsimp/pvcsumm.htm (12/9/99).

FTCBCP (Federal Trade Commission Bureau of Consumer Protection), 1995, "Nation's Largest Insurance Reporting Agency Agrees to Expand Consumer Rights," press release, June 21, http://www.ftc.gov/opa/9506/mib.htm (4/22/98).

Givens, Beth, 1997, "A Review of State and Federal Privacy Laws," San Diego, CA: Privacy Rights Clearinghouse, http://www. privacyrights.org (4/22/98).

Gostin, Lawrence O., 1995, "Health Information Privacy," *Cornell Law Review*, 80:451–528.

HLI (JRI Health Law Institute), 1996, "Whitepaper: U.S. Health Information Privacy Policy: Theory and Practice," http://www.jrihealth.org/programs/law/health_privacy.shtml (4/22/98).

JCAHO/NCQA (Joint Commission on Accreditation of Healthcare Organizations/National Committee for Quality Assurance), 1998, "Protecting Personal Health Information: A Framework for Meeting the Challenges in a Managed Care Environment," http://www.ncqa.org/pages/communications/news/tablcont.htm (4/14/99).

Krause, Micki, and Laura Brown, 1996, "Information Security in the Healthcare Industry," *Information Systems Security*, 5(3):32–41.

Merz, Jon F., Pamala Sankar, and Simon S. Yoo, 1998, "Hospital Consent for Disclosure of Medical Records," *Journal of Law, Medicine and Ethics*, 26(3):241–249.

Nagel, Denise, 1997, "Medical Privacy: An Opportunity for Innovative State Initiatives," Lexington, MA: National Coalition for Patients Rights, http://www.tiac.net/users/gls/cprne.html (4/22/98).

OTA (U.S. Congress, Office of Technology Assessment), 1993, Protecting Privacy in Computerized Medical Information, OTA-TCT-576, Washington, DC: U.S. Government Printing Office, http://www.wws.princeton.edu/cgi-bin/byteserv.prl/ota/disk1/1993/9342/9342.PDF (4/22/98).

Perrone, Janice, 1997, "Open Secrets," *Hospitals and Health Networks*, 71(21):68.

Pretzer, Michael, 1999, "The Clock Is Ticking on Patient Privacy," *Medical Economics*, 76(2):29–32.

Privacy Rights Clearinghouse, 1997, "Factsheet #8: How Private Is My Medical Information?" http://www.privacyrights.org/fs/fs8-med.html (4/22/98).

Siegler, Mark, 1999, "Confidentiality in Medicine—A Decrepit Concept," in Tom L. Beauchamp and LeRoy Walters, eds., *Contemporary Issues in Bioethics*, 5th ed., Belmont, CA: Wadsworth Publishing Company.

Silberner, Joanne, 1997, "Keeping Confidence," *Hastings Center Report*, 27(6):8.

Tarasoff (*Tarasoff v. Board of Regents*), 1976, 551 P2d 334.

Thompson, Dennis F., 1992, "Hospital Ethics," *Cambridge Quarterly of Healthcare Ethics*, 1(3):203–210.

8

PATIENT SERVICES

Before the Medicare prospective payment system was introduced in the early 1980s, hospitals were not greatly concerned about the amount of uncompensated care they provided. The cost of such care was shifted from patients who could not pay to those who could. The cost reimbursement system virtually assured healthcare organizations that they would be paid for care that was given, regardless of who received it. Hospitals could literally add up their total operating costs and divide the bill among the paying patients. When Medicare started paying fixed amounts according to DRGs, however, the costs of charity care could no longer be divided among the paying patients. When other payers followed the Medicare example with provider contracts and fee schedules, the pool of patients from whom the hospital's costs for uncompensated care could be recovered was reduced even further. Economic constraints now make it necessary for all healthcare organizations to watch very closely the amount of charity care they give.

PATIENT DUMPING

As it became increasingly difficult to shift the costs of nonpaying patients to those who were insured, some hospitals took the position that the provision of charity care was not their responsibility and began to send patients who had no means of paying to other hospitals (Annas, 1986; Spielman, 1988). In December 1986, for example, Mrs. Rosa Rivera arrived at the emergency room of DeTar Hospital in Victoria, Texas, in labor. She had received no prenatal care and had no health insurance. Because she did not have a private physician, she was assigned to Dr. Michael L. Burditt, who was next on DeTar's list of on-call obstetricians. When Burditt learned of Mrs. Rivera's financial situation, he told the nurse that he did not want to care for her and ordered her to be transferred to a public hospital 170 miles away. The nurse told Dr. Burditt that under federal regulations he would have to examine Mrs. Rivera before she could be transferred. He did examine her and found that she had dangerously high blood pressure, which could lead to serious complications during delivery. Nonetheless, Burditt signed a Physician's Certificate Authorizing Transfer without listing any reasons. Two hours later, an ambulance arrived for the transfer. Burditt did not order medication or life support equipment for Mrs. Rivera during the transfer. About 40 miles outside of Victoria, Mrs. Rivera gave birth. The nurse called Dr. Burditt, who ordered them to continue on to the public hospital. Mrs. Rivera wanted to return to DeTar, however. She was finally treated by another physician at DeTar and was released with her baby three days later (Burditt, 1991; Hylton, 1992)

The combination of rapidly increasing burdens on some public hospitals with a growing number of well-publicized stories of patient dumping such as the case of Mrs. Rivera prompted congressional action. Only three years after the establishment of the Medicare DRG system, the Consolidated Omnibus Budget Reconciliation Act of 1986 (COBRA) included a section known as the Emergency Medical Treatment and Active Labor Act (EMTALA), which established specific duties for all hospitals that participate in the Medicare program with respect to emergency care (Frew, 1997a). What was originally an ethical problem became a legal matter as well.

Briefly, hospitals now have the following requirements under EMTALA:

1. To provide medical screening examinations to all patients who present themselves and request care, regardless of their ability to pay. The law applies to all facilities that operate under a healthcare organization's Medicare provider number, including off-campus and nonemergency departments. *Examination* in this context means an examination by a physician or a physician's assistant and appropriate tests if indicated.

2. To provide stabilizing care so that the patient's condition will not deteriorate if her or she is transferred or discharged. In addition to trauma cases, a woman in active labor is not considered to be in a stable condition until the baby is delivered.

3. To treat unstable patients when the hospital has the capability and capacity to treat them. Unstable patients may be transferred only for reasons of medical necessity, that is, when the risks of transfer are outweighed by the anticipated benefits. Hospitals are not required to keep formal lists of their service capabilities (except under Florida state law), but they will be held to a disparate treatment standard. The fact that they treat paying patients in certain conditions constitutes proof that they are able to treat nonpaying patients in similar conditions.

4. To maintain a list of on-call physicians in every specialty privileged to practice in the hospital unless there are too few providers to cover certain services. The list is to be posted, and records are to be kept of who is on call at any given time. The hospital is required to report on-call physicians who do not respond to requests, and physicians as well as hospitals are subject to civil penalties for failure to treat medical emergencies.

5. To transfer patients only when medically necessary, only with the consent of the receiving hospital and the patient, and only by appropriately equipped vehicles with adequate attendant personnel. Receiving hospitals are required to accept medically necessary transfers when they have the capability to treat. A copy of the medical record must be sent with the patient.

The scope of the required medical examinations for emergency patients has been specified in detail in advisory communications from the Health Care Financing Administration and in case rulings (Frew, 1997b). The term *emergency medical condition (EMC)* has been the subject of considerable debate, however, because the COBRA definition differed from that used by the American College of Emergency Physicians (Rosenstein, 1993). According to the statute, an EMC is

> A medical condition manifesting itself by acute symptoms of sufficient severity (including severe pain) such that the absence of immediate medical attention could reasonably be expected to result in:
> a. .placing the health of the individual (or, with respect to a pregnant woman, the health of the woman or her unborn child) in serious jeopardy,
> b. serious impairment to bodily functions, or
> c. serious dysfunction of any bodily organ or part, or, with respect to a pregnant woman who is having contractions:
> (a) that there is inadequate time to effect a safe transfer to another hospital before delivery, or
> (b) that the transfer may pose a threat to the health or safety of the woman or her unborn child.
>
> (Fosmire, 1996)

The distinction between an inadequate medical examination and a misdiagnosis can be very difficult to make (Summers, 1996). Other terms in the law, such as *serious impairment* and *active labor* are equally imprecise. The intent of the law, however, is clear: EMTALA is directed to disparate treatment between paying and nonpaying patients. "Probably the single most important thing a hospital can do," according to Charlotte Yeh and Nancy Trombly, writing in the newsletter of the Harvard Risk Management Foundation, "is to have—and follow—a consistent, non-discriminatory process for screening and transfer of individuals who come to the [emergency department] seeking care" (Yeh and Trombly, 1997; see also Wood, 1996).

The EMTALA has been criticized for its weak enforcement provisions. The maximum fine ($50,000) may be too low to deter patient dumping, and the threat of Medicare decertification is so severe a penalty that it has been imposed only when patient dumping was accompanied by other Medicare violations (Hylton, 1992). The stabilization requirement, furthermore, doesn't prevent dumping but only limits it (Hall, 1988). It has also been noted that the COBRA regulatory approach addresses the immediate problem of patient dumping without touching on the underlying cause: the 18% of the population that has no health insurance (Hylton, 1992; Rosenstein, 1993).

Healthcare administrators and ethics committees are faced with a number of problems that arise in connection with the provision of emergency care under EMTALA. These include treating noncompliant patients such as alcohol and drug abusers, training staff members to meet EMTALA requirements while dealing with patients and their families in crisis situations, and obtaining adequate documentation from physicians for refusals of treatment and medically appropriate transfers.

One area that often raises ethical questions is the relationship between emergency departments and MCOs. Understandably, MCOs do not want their plan members going to emergency rooms when they should be seen at physicians' offices or clinics. They may therefore refuse to authorize payment for emergency care; in fact, MCOs may take advantage of the situation if they know that the hospital is required by law to provide the care whether it gets paid or not. Why should the MCO pay if the hospital is required to provide the service anyway? Congress addressed this issue with a provision in the 1997 Balanced Budget Act that requires managed care plans to pay for emergency care for plan members if a "prudent layperson" could reasonably expect that his or her health was in jeopardy. The law is not settled on this issue, however, and coordination problems between MCOs and emergency departments will still have to be worked out.

Another area in which emergency department administrators face ethical decisions is the *snitch rule* (Fosmire, 1996). Hospitals on the receiving end of patient dumping are generally the only parties that can provide actual evidence that a transfer was inappropriate. Receiving hospitals, however, have been reluctant to report violations. They often have established relationships with the hospitals that transfer nonpaying patients and rely on them for other referrals. During the first few years after COBRA was passed, there were very few reports of inappropriate transfers and, because adequate evidence was difficult to obtain, even fewer cases that went beyond the initial investigation stage (Hylton, 1992). The HCFA therefore issued a regulation requiring participating hospitals "to report to HCFA or the State survey agency any time it has reason to believe it may have received an individual who has been transferred in an unstable emergency medical condition from another hospital in violation of Section 489.24(d)" (HCFA, 1994).

This snitch rule has apparently helped. In the first ten years after the passage of COBRA, the Department of Health and Human Services cited only 503 hospitals for violations and penalized only 41 providers. Under the new rule, the pace of enforcement has picked up dramatically. According to a 1997 Public Citizen's Health Research Group report:

> Between April 1, 1995 and September 30, 1996, DHHS identified 256 hospitals responsible for 264 dumping violations. Twenty-three of these hospitals (9 percent) had been cited for prior violations. In addition, in 1995 and 1996, the Office of Inspector General (OIG), the agency within DHHS with the authority to impose fines for patient dumping violations, concluded settlements with 26 hospitals and eight doctors, where the hospitals or doctors paid a fine to resolve a complaint of patient dumping. . . . Twenty-five of the twenty-six hospital agreements include "community outreach" provisions, describing steps the hospital promises to take to publicize its availability to treat emergency patients, regardless of their ability to pay.
>
> (Public Citizen, 1997)

The ethical issues involved in charity care and patient dumping extend well beyond the matter of legal compliance, however. Whether a hospital has been transferring patients in unstable conditions may be determined on the basis of a pattern of practice rather than a single incident, so the decision to report a transferring hospital is still likely to involve difficult aspects of provider relations, responsibility to the community, and other stakeholder interests. Healthcare organizations need to determine for themselves the extent of their obligation to emergency patients and to their communities based on an ethical analysis of their own goals and the needs of their many stakeholders. The American Public Health Association addressed this matter in a 1988 resolution urging private and public hospitals to "adopt policies that no emergency patients be transferred for non-medical reasons even after being stabilized" (APHA, 1988).

Case 8.1 Christopher Sercye

On May 18, 1998, Cable News Network carried the following story:

> *Just outside hospital, teen lay bleeding to death*
> *Workers cite policy in refusal to help*
>
> CHICAGO (CNN)—A 15-year-old boy lay bleeding to death just outside a hospital while emergency room workers refused to help, citing a policy preventing them

from going outside. Christopher Sercye was shot Saturday while playing basketball just steps away from Ravenswood Hospital. His friends managed to drag him to within a few feet of the hospital's entrance, but workers refused to help—even though friends, neighbors and police pleaded with them. Actually, Sercye was still alive when, 25 minutes after the shooting, a police officer finally commandeered a wheelchair and took him inside. It was too late. A bullet had perforated his aorta, and Sercye died about an hour after being brought inside. Late Monday, John E. Blair, the hospital's president and chief executive officer, announced that Ravenswood had rescinded the policy that prevented employees from going outside to help Sercye.

"I have instructed my staff to provide treatment to anyone who needs it in the immediate vicinity of the hospital when there are no paramedics or medical technicians available," Blair said in a written statement. "Above all, I want to make sure that if a tragedy like this ever occurs again, we have a different result." Blair had previously said the hospital was reviewing its policies and that it was not equipped to deal with trauma cases like gunshot wounds.

(CNN, 1998)

The problem raised here is one of determining the limits of the obligation to offer care. Individuals caught in tragic situations and local communities have a right to expect that healthcare organizations will offer assistance. Formulating an institutional policy to cover this type of emergency, however, is no easy matter. If staff members leave hospital property to rescue someone, how far should they go? The staff available to offer assistance, furthermore, may not be trained for the emergency service that is needed. Requests may also occur in situations where there is great risk—for example, if an assailant is still present.

DISCHARGE PLANNING

Some of the most difficult cases for administrators and direct caregivers involve discharge planning. One clinical/organizational ethics committee, for example, was asked to see a woman with a number of health problems, including the effects of a stroke, diabetes, and Crohn's disease. She had been in and out of the hospital almost every month for a year. She was in a wheelchair and could not take care of herself at home very well. Her husband was receiving disability checks, but he also worked regular hours at a minimum-wage job. At times, when the patient was afraid to stay home alone, she went with her husband and stayed in his pickup truck while he worked. They had two adult children. One held two jobs to support her family and could not care for her mother; the other, a son, flatly refused to help and said he could not stand to be in the same room with his father. Placement in a day-care program three days a week helped for a while, but continuation of this care would have required an application for Medicaid. The patient's condition was such that she could have been placed in a long-term care facility and would have been eligible for Medicaid. The patient was not the problem; she was a very pleasant person and certainly appreciative of the care she received—always eager, in fact, to return to the emergency room. Her husband, however, was afraid he would lose his house if she became Medicaid dependent (which was not true) and that his disability checks would be discontinued if the state found out that he was working (which probably was true). At any rate, he refused to apply for Medicaid. The case came to the ethics committee when the discharge planner had run out of alternatives and was growing short on patience. The husband absolutely refused to accept the appropriate placement, and the patient was periodically readmitted through the emergency room when her condition deteriorated. The ethics committee met with the patient and her family—except for her son—and more or less pressured the husband into agreeing to apply for Medicaid so that the woman could be placed in a nursing home. Some members of the committee felt that the committee was being used by the hospital to force a patient into compliance, even though they were in complete agreement that discharge to a nursing home was in the patient's best interest. The Medicaid application was held up at the state level, however, and the husband changed his mind before the placement could be completed. The patient was eventually discharged home, but she was hospitalized through the emergency department again three weeks later. The social worker refused to have her "discharged to the truck," and the husband refused to meet again with the ethics committee. The hospital in this case accepted its moral obligation to do what was best for the patient, but rules and policies made it difficult to find an acceptable solution.

Effective discharge planning has been one of the major requirements for accreditation by the JCAHO for many years. In 1997, the HCFA required Medicare providers to develop discharge plans for all patients. The plans must include a patient evaluation that addresses the need for posthospital care and arrangements for the initial implementation of the plan (DHHS, 1997). The HCFA regulations were then supplemented by requirements in the Balanced Budget Act of 1997. Hospitals had been actively channeling discharge patients to subsidiary or financially related long-term care facilities and advising patients to select hospital-related home health agency services. Congress was concerned that this self-dealing would restrict patient choice. The Balanced Budget Act now requires hospitals to give each patient a list of Medicare-certified providers of home health care that serve the patient's area. The act also requires that

> the discharge plan shall (i) not specify or otherwise limit the qualified provider which may provide post-hospital home health services, and (ii) identify . . . any entity to whom the individual is referred in which the hospital has a disclosable financial interest . . . or which has an interest in the hospital.
>
> (HCFA, 1997)

Beginning in August 1998, hospitals were also required to disclose the nature of their financial interest in any home health or other postacute services to the

HCFA, along with data on the percentage of discharged individuals who received services from hospital-affiliated providers (42 USC 1395x(ee)).

These are reasonable regulations for assuring patients the right to select providers, but they pose certain problems for hospital administrators. Keeping an accurate list of currently Medicare-certified home health care providers in the hospital's service area is not a problem, but providing a similar list to patients who may come from other areas—or from across the country—can be more difficult. The question of recommendations is even more problematic. The JCAHO accreditation standards require hospitals to give advice to patients and their families regarding the ability of various agencies to provide the type of care needed when the patient is discharged (JCAHO, 1996). The HCFA regulations, however, appear to prohibit hospitals from giving explicit recommendations. The requirement that the hospital "not specify or otherwise limit" the providers on the list given to a patient is at best vague and at worst in conflict with any effort to give patients sound advice. Whether a discharge nurse or social worker is permitted to answer patients' questions about the services or the quality of different providers is a matter of interpretation. Simply offering patients a list of providers may also raise the question of whether the hospital is actually recommending the providers on the list. The AHA has recommended that hospitals include a disclaimer to the effect that being included on the list does not constitute a recommendation or endorsement by the hospital (AHA, 1998). Problems associated with discharge procedures may also fall under the purview of a clinical ethics committee, such as the question of a referral for aggressive treatment when, in the judgment of the physician, the patient is clearly terminal and palliative measures would be more appropriate.

ETHICAL PERSPECTIVES

Patient care is always a matter of fitting the individual with his or her unique needs into the pattern of services that the healthcare organization provides. Ethically, this is a matter of human rights, as outlined in Chapter 1. Respect for people as individuals requires that one take account of their unique conditions and needs. This means that the organization is obligated to value every person with respect to his or her individual differences. This duty, however, is often overridden by what are presumed to be organizational necessities. Organizations by nature must provide services according to rules and procedures specifying what will or will not be provided, what can and cannot be offered, and who will do it. There is certainly some sense to this. Organizations, as the German sociologist Max Weber explained, are necessarily bureaucratic: they can attain the efficiency needed to serve the number of people in their charge only by having set procedures and guidelines. Such policies and procedures, however, inevitably overlook the differences and special needs that distinguish people as individuals. The ethical responsibility to respect these individual differences cannot be set aside for purely bureaucratic reasons or because of a perception of some organizational necessity. Although healthcare organizations take greater account of individual differences than many other organizations, there are still points at which the procedural rules of the organization must be adjusted to accommodate the needs of individuals.

This obligation is especially evident in the professional standards of the people providing direct patient care. The healthcare professional, by definition, has a duty to the patient as well as to the organization for which he or she works. This is the great merit of our professional system. But it implies that professionals who work in organizational settings will find themselves on the boundary between the interests of the organization and the rights of individual patients. Professionals do have a dual responsibility of patient advocacy and loyalty to the organizations for which they work, but they cannot allow the latter to override the former by deferring to organizational demands at the expense of their patients.

Many healthcare organizational mission statements, of course, claim that individual patient care is paramount. This principle, however, is only as good as its implementation. Effective implementation of a commitment to patient care requires organizations to have sufficient respect for the professional standards of their caregivers to ensure that these professionals have the power and the resources to take actions that meet the needs of their patients. A commitment to patient care implies respect and support for those people whose professional activity places them at the boundary between the organizations they work for and the individuals they serve.

The ethical responsibility to respect individual needs is especially evident in social work practice (Blumenfield and Lowe, 1987). The first words of the Code of Ethics of the National Association of Social Workers (NASW) mention the obligation of client advocacy:

> The primary mission of the social work profession is to enhance human well-being and help meet the basic human needs of all people, with particular attention to the needs and empowerment of people who are vulnerable, oppressed, and living in poverty.
>
> (NASW, 1997)

The NASW Code acknowledges, however, that this commitment can come into conflict with the organizations that employ social workers, and it insists that the commitment to the patient must not be abandoned:

> Instances may arise when social workers' ethical obligations conflict with agency policies or relevant laws or regulations. When such conflicts occur, social workers must make a responsible effort to resolve the conflict in a manner that is consistent with the values, principles, and standards expressed in this Code.
>
> (NASW, 1997)

The inevitable conflict involved in this boundary situation is recognized in law in several states. In North Carolina, for example, the law supports the social worker's role as client advocate even when confronted with organizational pressures:

> As employees of institutions or agencies, social workers are responsible for remaining alert to and attempting to moderate institutional pressures or policies that conflict with the standards of their profession. If such conflict arises, social workers' responsibility shall be to uphold the ethical standards of their profession.
>
> (North Carolina, 1991)

The NASW Code of Ethics raises another ethical issue of this boundary situation: the responsibility of social work professionals to be advocates for social justice within the organizations for which they work. According to the Code, "Social workers pursue social change, particularly with and on behalf of vulnerable and oppressed individuals and groups of people" (NASW, 1997). Healthcare organizations must be responsive to the efforts of professionals to improve policies and procedures (see Beck et al., 1993).

The obligations of healthcare professionals with regard to patient services can also be viewed from the stakeholder perspective. Patients clearly have a stake in the services they receive, but it is not always recognized that healthcare professionals who are obligated to be advocates for their patients have a stake in providing these services effectively. Nor is it always recognized that healthcare administrators, for whom the interests of the organization are paramount, have an obligation to provide effective services to patients—an obligation that puts them in a boundary situation similar to that of direct service professionals. The ideal, from the stakeholder perspective, is to attain a comprehensive vision of the organization so that the interests of participants coincide more than they conflict. The particular interests of administrators in patient care will become more apparent in the discussion of the business aspects of patient services below. But first consider the interplay of stakeholder interests, professional responsibilities, and organizational goals in the following case.

Case 8.2 Medical Futility

Mrs. Adkins was admitted to St. Vincent de Paul Hospital for a hip replacement after a fall. She had been reasonably healthy despite her diabetes, which had led to poor circulation in her extremities and signs of necrotic tissue in her left toes. She was 83 years old and lived with her son. She had two daughters and one sister with whom she attended the Free Will Baptist Church, where her brother-in-law was an associate pastor. Mrs. Adkins' husband had died 12 years earlier, and she still received his pension from the steel mill along with her Social Security benefits. Her son, Michael, worked for the mill as well, but was laid off 18 months before her hospitalization with the promise of being called back when market conditions improved.

The surgery was successful, but Mrs. Adkins did not tolerate the anesthesia very well. She was nauseous when she tried to sit up and could not get out of bed. Three days after the operation, Mrs. Adkins suffered a stroke. She aspirated some food, causing an obstruction, and an emergency tracheostomy was necessary. She was placed on a ventilator. She lost consciousness for about four hours during this episode and was disoriented when she revived. After the stroke, her condition deteriorated rapidly. When she was conscious she was disoriented, and her periods of consciousness became shorter and less frequent. Brain activity continued to decline. The neurologist believed that the events associated with the stroke had cut off the oxygen to her brain long enough to do irreversible damage. A feeding tube was placed a week later for nutrition. Dialysis was started two weeks after the stroke. After three weeks, no upper-brain activity was evident.

Mrs. Adkins remained in this condition without further incident for the next four weeks. The attending physician was quite frank about her poor prognosis in discussions with her son, one daughter, and Mrs. Adkins' sister. The family remained hopeful, however, despite the fact that the attending physician and the neurologist gave them no encouragement. "We just can't give up," her son said. "She would never have wanted us to give up. She believed in God and always believed that if we just kept our faith, things would turn out all right." Michael believed that this was God's way of testing him and that if he did not give up on his mother, God would "send her back." Since she was no longer conscious, he visited less frequently.

By the sixth week, Mrs. Adkins showed no signs of consciousness and the staff began to feel that the situation was hopeless and should not be permitted to continue. The gangrene, which remained dry, had spread through her left foot, and signs of necrosis appeared in her right foot. The physician, the neurologist, and the hospital chaplain met with the family. After much discussion, the son acquiesced to the physician's request for permission to write an order not to resuscitate, but he would not consider withdrawal of life support. He asked if amputation would be appropriate for the left foot, but the doctor said that the gangrene was not spreading through the patient's body at this point.

Since Mrs. Adkins' condition was stable, transfer to a nursing home was considered. The level of care required, however, was not available in the area. The nearest facility that could care for a patient in her condition was 145 miles away and could not accept her at the time. Since there were no other alternatives available, the social worker suggested a consultation with the ethics committee. The son flatly rejected this offer, saying that this was just a way to force him into giving up on his mother. He then refused to talk further with the social worker. At the request of the physician and the social worker, the ethics committee considered the case and asked the chaplain to intervene. The chaplain found the son's attitude to be much the same as it had been during the earlier conference with the attending physician and the neurologist. He contacted Mrs. Adkins' brother-in-law for assistance. The brother-in-law (Mrs. Adkins' pastor) said that he had personally advised her children to discontinue treatment and allow Mrs. Adkins to die peacefully. The chaplain then spoke to Mrs. Adkins' daughter. Her position was that she would consider withdrawing the ventilator and stopping the dialysis, but that she could never make a decision concerning her mother without her brother's agreement. She felt that the family must "stick together" at this difficult time.

At a subsequent ethics committee meeting, a social worker raised the issue of the cost of this futile care. The committee was informed that Medicare would not cover Mrs. Adkins' care after about the sixth week. After that time, the hospital would have to bear the cost of Mrs. Adkins' continued care. One committee member said that he considered this to be a waste of community resources. "Patients and their families should not have unlimited access to resources that could be better used for other people," he said.

Concerned that this state of affairs was wrong both for the patient and in light of the hospital's mission, the ethics committee asked the social worker to write to the patient's son indicating that he would have to accept responsibility for planning for his mother's care. The social worker drafted a letter outlining the available alternatives, including hospice care, and informing the family that Mrs. Adkins would be responsible for the cost of her care at the hospital when her Medicare coverage was exhausted. The letter was viewed as an effort to initiate a planning process, but the ethics committee really did not know how far the hospital should go in terms of putting pressure on the family if it insisted on maintaining the status quo. The committee was aware of institutional futile care policies establishing procedures that can lead to a discontinuation of treatment without the consent of the family (Halevy and Brody, 1996; Johnson and Potter, 1997), but it was reluctant to recommend the use of such policies.

The issue of medical futility is a serious concern for physicians, but it is even more of a concern for healthcare administrators (Orr and Gensen, 1997; Zucker and Zucker, 1997). Physicians can maintain patients in nonprogressive conditions for a long time; healthcare administrators have staff morale and the efficient use of public resources to consider. Transfer and reimbursement are primarily organizational problems, not medical issues. The hospital in this case had a continuing responsibility to Mrs. Adkins. Whether an institution should ever adopt a position that life-sustaining treatment should be withdrawn is debatable. It has a prima facie duty to support the position taken by the physician, but some physicians insist on offering heroic measures and others simply do not want to challenge family decisions.

Administrators, however, have other issues to consider. Most of the staff responsible for Mrs. Adkins' daily care felt that it was wrong to continue this futile treatment; their conscientious objections to what they were doing had to be considered. Since there was no longer any effective treatment available for Mrs. Adkins, she should have been moved to another level of care. Organizational resources also had to be considered. When third-party payments were exhausted, the hospital would have to charge the patient directly (with little hope that it would be paid) or accept the cost itself. Reasonable people may disagree about this, but I would say that the family must take its share of the responsibility. They should be informed about the cost of the care they are requesting and the patient's responsibility for it.

While it should be obvious that healthcare organizations must be careful about devoting community resources to care that is medically inappropriate, my opinion on this matter appears to differ from the position taken by the JCAHO. An exemplary standard in the "Organizational Ethics" section of the JCAHO *Manual* states that

> Admission and transfer policies are not based on patient or hospital economics. Only patients whose specific condition or disease cannot be safely treated at the hospital are diverted, refused admission, or transferred to another hospital.
>
> (JCAHO, 1996)

Practical solutions to the problem of futile care will, I believe, call this standard into question. At the organizational level, economic issues cannot be avoided.

PRICING

The conventional wisdom has been that health care is so important that the physician should do whatever the patient needs, regardless of the cost. This was

certainly common practice in the past, and it helped promote the rampant inflation of healthcare costs and the extraordinary expansion of the healthcare sector
that took place between the 1960s and the 1980s. When the federal health
planning program of the 1970s failed to stem the tide, Medicare resorted to
price controls. Healthcare administrators were then among the first to become
cost conscious. Now treatment approvals, fee schedules, and other controls are
being imposed by all payers, and we are well into a provider contract frenzy
that involves physicians and staff professionals.

Except for the pharmaceutical industry, competitive pricing had not been
much of a concern to healthcare organizations in the past. As the healthcare
sector moves closer to price competition, however, healthcare administrators
need to exercise greater care. Abusive business practices such as deceptive
pricing and undue influence that takes advantage of vulnerable patients are illegal under federal law. As insurance policies, managed care plan contracts, and
agreements for home health and other services become more complicated,
claims of deceptive practice can be expected to increase.

While direct conspiracies to fix prices are not very common, some practices
have been judged to be illegally anticompetitive. In 1982 the state of Arizona
brought a case against the Maricopa County Medical Society challenging a
contractual plan that set price limits for specific services. The Maricopa County
Medical Society, of which 70% of the physicians practicing in the county were
members, attempted to develop its own fee schedule so that it could bargain
with insurance companies, employers, and health plans. By a four to three vote,
the U.S. Supreme Court found that such an agreement was a violation of the
Sherman Antitrust Act (Maricopa, 1982). This effort to carve out an exemption
for healthcare organizations under antitrust laws failed. Healthcare organizations need to be mindful of antitrust implications of the many new types of
contractual arrangements they may consider.

A 1994 opinion from the secretary of the FTC addressed a number of related
points (FTC, 1994). The AMA and the Chicago Medical Society had requested
approval of a program for review of physicians' fees. The FTC found that the
Medical Society could establish a grievance committee to which patients could
complain concerning unreasonable fees, provision of unnecessary services, and
exerting undue influence on vulnerable patients. The FTC opinion also stated
that medical societies could "adopt an across-the-board requirement that physicians disclose relevant fee information in advance of treatment whenever it is
possible to do so, just as they currently require physicians to disclose in advance the possible risks of treatment in order to obtain informed consent to the
treatment" (FTC, 1994). The FTC did not permit medical societies to determine
that certain fee levels amounted to "fee gouging," however, since this would
constitute a form of price fixing.

As health care becomes more competitive, providers may be tempted to attempt to corner a market by driving out competitors. The effort to drive out competition through predatory pricing is illegal under both federal law and many state laws (Shils, 1997). In 1993 the mega-retail discount chain Wal-Mart was sued for selling drugs and health and beauty aids below cost at its store in Conway, Arkansas. Three local pharmacies accused Wal-Mart of violating the Arkansas state law against predatory pricing. The Chancery Court awarded them $300,000 in damages and ordered Wal-Mart to stop the practice (Arkansas, 1993), but the decision was reversed on appeal (Wal-Mart, 1995; see also Shils, 1997). Although predatory pricing has not been common in health care, competition in the managed care market—where companies must have a membership of a certain size to be viable—and even among hospitals in regions where there may be too many facilities for all to prosper may tempt organizations to consider such techniques.

Other questions about pricing may be of concern in view of the organizational mission. Organizations should consider whether services that are especially beneficial can be priced within an affordable range for uninsured people, whether services that are typically not covered by insurance can be offered at lower prices, and whether charges for some basic services can be put on a sliding scale relative to household income.

Case 8.3 Cost Shifting

The question of pricing also raises the issue of cost shifting. In one respect, cost shifting is universal and unavoidable. As long as there are patients who cannot or will not pay their bills, the cost will be shifted to some other payer. With discounts, contractual allowances, and new federal regulations in place, however, cost shifting in medical centers, hospitals, and clinics has become a complicated matter. The following case was written by Dr. Donald Pathoff, DDS, FACD:

> One common procedure in oral surgery is the setting of fractured jaws. The closed reduction procedure for setting a fractured mandible is typical. This procedure is normally done in a dentist's office, but for more difficult cases, for patients with other medical complications, and sometimes for children or at the patient's request, the procedure can be done at a hospital. Let us assume that the normal charges associated with the procedure done in the office or at the hospital are as follows:
>
> | | Hospital | Office |
> | --- | --- | --- |
> | Operating room | $1000 | — |
> | Recovery room | 300 | — |
> | Anesthetist | 650 | 400 |
> | Supplies | 300 | — |
> | Surgery fee | 2000 | 2000 |
> | Hospital visit | 175 | — |
> | Consultant | 75 | — |

A dentist can raise the surgery fee to $2500 for complex cases. Because of the time involved, however, it is generally more profitable to do these procedures in the office.

Now let us assume that the following four patients require closed reduction mandible jaw reconstruction:

- Patient A, a 40-year-old self-employed carpenter, was injured at work. He can pay the full charges, but only on an extended payment plan.
- Patient B, a 61-year-old ex-custodian, suffered a broken jaw in a fall. Because of complications, the best reconstruction could be done in the hospital. It is unlikely that he will be able to pay at all, even though he willingly promised the receptionist that he would pay. At the hospital he would qualify for charity care.
- Patient C, a 52-year-old telephone company executive, was in a traffic accident. His insurance is through a managed care plan. The procedure approval clerk said that the plan will pay $1600 for the surgery, but the operation can only be approved as an office procedure.
- Patient D, a 45-year-old lawyer, was injured accidentally by his golf partner. This is the least urgent of the four cases, but there are some minor complications with the reconstruction, and the patient wants the best care possible. At his request, the procedure would be done at the hospital. He has very good indemnity insurance coverage; it would pay the normal surgical charges or the higher rate for a more complicated procedure.

Let us assume further that all of these patients have been referred to an oral surgeon by other doctors or dentists. The surgeon has earned the respect of the medical community and is reluctant to refuse any referrals. He would normally bill each patient at his customary rate. The question is whether he will get paid what he charges or write off portions of some of the bills as charity. Patient B probably won't pay at all. Patient A will eventually pay the full charges. The managed care plan paying for patient C does not pay at a rate sufficient to allow the surgeon to recoup much of his losses on other patients. This means that the cost of treating patient B will be paid by patient D's insurance and by patient A.

Is this sort of cost shifting unethical? It may seem initially that shifting the cost from patient B to patients D and A is unfair. This has been an established practice in American health care for decades, however. The participants in a 1994 seminar convened by the Woodstock Theological Center found such cost shifting generally acceptable.

> Charges to full-paying patients have traditionally helped to cover some of the costs of those unable to pay. While this practice also raises fairness questions, in the absence of some form of universal health care coverage, members of the [Woodstock] group believe it to be an ethically defensible practice, as long as the extra income from paying patients is committed to providing services to individuals who cannot pay.
>
> (Woodstock, 1995:17)

Other commentators, however, find this temporary fix to be seriously flawed (Patthoff, personal communication). It only works until the cost-shifting loopholes are closed, and it can give the false impression that those who pay less are actually paying the full cost.

To whom would the cost shifting be most unfair, however? When it is shifted to patient D, it is actually shifted to all people insured under his plan. When it is shifted to patient A, it is shifted to him personally. Should the surgeon offer a discount to patient

A? His professional guidelines call for charging all customers at the same rate. But if public clinics can charge customers on a sliding scale relative to household income, why shouldn't he do the same by offering to forgive part of the bill for a particular patient? And why should the managed care plan escape the cost shifting?

BILLING AND COLLECTIONS

In the section on "Organizational Ethics" of its 1997 *Accreditation Manual*, the JCAHO states that hospitals should have a "code of ethical behavior" that addresses billing. The Commission's explanation is brief but includes the following statement of standards:

> All patient billing is itemized and includes dates of service. The hospital has a formal process to review patient or other payer questions about charges expeditiously and resolve a conflict or discuss a question without real or perceived harassment.
>
> (JCAHO, 1996:RI-24)

Patients have a right to receive itemized bills for hospital care, long-term care, home health care, and other services. Whether patients can understand their hospital bills is another matter. In fact, concerns over billing may be the single point at which customers become most upset with healthcare providers. If the development of long-term relationships with customers is a marketing goal for a healthcare organization, customer hospitality in financial dealings (i.e., clearer bills and full explanations) is a must. This is another area in which good organizational ethics is good business.

Healthcare organizations should, of course, get paid for their services. In the past not-for-profit hospitals were reluctant to pursue collections aggressively for a number of reasons. First, they realized that there are some people who just cannot pay. But hospitals were also understandably reluctant to risk bad publicity by pressing claims too vigorously. One result of this reluctance, however, was that some people who could afford to pay simply refused to do so, knowing that little or no action would be taken against them. This situation is changing now under increased financial pressures, but many hospitals are still reluctant to be aggressive with collections.

Not-for-profit hospitals usually send bills to patients for a period of six months to a year. If there is no effort to pay or to make arrangements to pay, they send the bill to a collection agency. If there is still no response, the bill comes back and is often sent to another agency. This can be expensive because the hospital will have to pay the collection agency 25% or more of whatever is collected. If the bill comes back uncollected, the hospital may report the customer to a credit bureau or it may initiate legal action. If it is thought that the person is unable to pay the bill, the hospital may just write it off as bad debt.

Healthcare organizations must also keep a watchful eye on the practices of their collection agencies. Agencies with better collection records may use techniques that harm the reputation of the healthcare organization, abuse valued customers, or are illegal. Ethically, it is as wrong to hire someone to do something immoral as it is to do it oneself. The federal Fair Debt Collections Practices Act sets limits on the activities of debt collectors. Common complaints received by the FTC include invasion of privacy, abusive language (including racial and ethnic slurs and sexual comments), communicating with relatives or friends about debts, and threats of jail or job loss (FTC, 1997). Debt collectors are not permitted to contact people at work without permission; they are required to submit itemized bills, and they cannot misrepresent themselves as lawyers or police officers (Azcuenaga, 1994). In 1997 the FTC reported taking action against such agencies as National Financial Services, Trans-Continental Affiliates, G & L Financial Services, United Creditor's Alliance Corporation, and Lundgren and Associates. The 1997 report to Congress contains the following note:

> Complaints concerning medical and hospital debts are becoming more evident. Some consumers allege that they never receive a final statement from the medical service provider and their accounts are forwarded, without further notice, to collection agencies which attempt to charge exorbitant interest, late fees and other collection costs in addition to the original debt. Some of these charges can exceed the debt itself.
>
> (FTC, 1997)

The billing and collection process involves a conflict of moral values. The collection program should be strong enough to require people who can afford it to pay their bills. But if it is insensitive to the fact that there are people who cannot pay, this may well be inconsistent with the public mission of the institution. Charting a middle course can be difficult.

CONCLUSIONS

While it is clear that organizational goals should encompass the best available service to patients and that patients should be given priority as primary stakeholders, the implementation of these moral commitments requires policies and procedures that are continually adjusted to patients' needs and to the professional standards of those who are responsible for direct services. An organizational code of conduct should address these patient service issues with appropriate standards. All who act on behalf of the organization should be required to assure that no one in need of emergency care will be turned away and that no one will be discharged without a plan that will safeguard his or her welfare. The organization should also provide complete and clear billing information using only accepted methods of calculating charges, and it should remain open and fair in resolving disputes. Reasonable disclosure of organizational financial interests and provider arrangements should be made.

With recent developments in healthcare financing and administration, economic realities are exercising much greater influence on patient care. This influence cannot be ignored. Efforts to avoid financial considerations will simply put the forces that are now driving the system out of the range of ethical consideration. If the ethical implications of these administrative and financial aspects are not explicitly addressed, the consequences will distort the pursuit of organizational goals and the fair treatment of all stakeholders.

REFERENCES

AHA (American Hospital Association), 1998, "Regulatory Advocacy Comment Letters, January 16, 1998," http://www.aha.org/ar/1–26.html (5/12/98).

Annas, George J., 1986, "Your Money or Your Life: 'Dumping' Uninsured Patients from Hospital Emergency Wards," *American Journal of Public Health*, 76(1):74–77.

APHA (American Public Health Association), 1988, "The Denial of Emergency Care to Uninsured Patients," *American Journal of Public Health*, 78(2):190.

Arkansas, 1993, Arkansas Chancery Court., Faulkner County: No. E-92-1158 (11 October 1993), reprinted in *Antitrust and Trade Regulation Report*, 65:541.

Azcuenaga, Mary L., 1994, "The Fair Debt Collection Practices Act at the Federal Trade Commission," http://www.ftc.gov/speeches/azcuenaga/cac94.htm (3/14/98).

Beck, Lasca, Barbara K. Miller, and Donna Adams, 1993, "Use of the Code of Ethics for Accountability in Discharge Planning," *Nursing Forum*, 28(3):5–12.

Blumenfield, Susan, and Jane Isaacs Lowe, 1987, "A Template for Analyzing Ethical Dilemmas in Discharge Planning," *Health and Social Work*, 12(1):47–56.

Burditt (*Burditt v. United States Department of Health and Human Services*), 1991, 934 F.2d 1362, 1366 (5th Cir. 1991).

CNN (Cable News Network), 1998, "Just Outside Hospital, Teen Lay Bleeding to Death," http://www.cnn.co.jp/US/9805/18/unhelpful.hospital (12/4/99).

DHHS (Department of Health and Human Services, Health Care Finance Administration), 1997, "State Operations Manual: Provider Certification, Transmittal No. 280," http://www.dischargedirect.com/HCFA_Memorandum.htm (5/3/98).

Fosmire, M. Sean, 1996, "Frequently Asked Questions about the Emergency Medical Treatment and Active Labor Act (EMTALA)," http://www.emtala.com (4/30/98).

Frew, Stephen, 1997a, "COBRA/EMTALA Online," Rockford, IL: Frew Consulting Group, http://www.medlaw.com (4/29/98).

——, 1997b, "COBRA/EMTALA Resources: Executive Summary," Rockford, IL: Frew Consulting Group, http://www.medlaw.com/handout.htm (4/29/98).

FTC (Federal Trade Commission), 1994, "American Medical Association—Advisory Opinion 009," February 14, 1994, http://www.ftc.gov/bc/adops/009.htm (5/17/99).

——, 1997, "Nineteenth Annual Report to Congress Pursuant to Section 815(a) of the

Fair Debt Collection Practices Act," http://www.ftc.gov/os/9703/fdcpa19s.htm (3/15/98).

Halevy, Amir, and Baruch A. Brody, 1996, "A Multi-institutional Collaborative Policy on Medical Futility," *Journal of the American Medical Association*, 276(7):571–574.

Hall, Mark, 1988, "The Unlikely Case in Favor of Patient Dumping," *Jurimetrics Journal*, 28:389–397.

HCFA (Department of Health and Human Services: Health Care Finance Administration), 1994, 42 CFR 489.20(m).

——, 1997, "Non-Discrimination in Post-Hospital Referral to Home Health Agencies and Other Entities (Balanced Budget Act of 1997, PL 103–55," http://www.dischargedirect.com/hcfa.htm (5/3/98).

HDM (Healthcare Data Management, Inc.), 1998, "Hospital/Medical Bill Recovery," http://healthaudit.com/auditmain.html (3/7/98).

Hylton, Maria O'Brien, 1992, "The Economics and Politics of Emergency Health Care for the Poor: The Patient Dumping Dilemma," *Brigham Young University Law Review*, 1992(4):971–1034.

JCAHO (Joint Commission on Accreditation of Healthcare Organizations), 1996, *Comprehensive Accreditation Manual for Hospitals: The Official Handbook. Refreshed Core, January 1998*, Oakbrook Terrace, IL: Joint Commission on Accreditation of Healthcare Organizations.

Johnson, Linda, and Robert Lyman Potter, 1997, "Professional and Public Community Projects for Developing Medical Futility Guidelines," in Marjorie B. Zucker, and Howard D. Zucker, eds., *Medical Futility and the Evolution of Life-Sustaining Interventions*, Cambridge, UK: Cambridge University Press.

Maricopa, 1982, *Arizona v. Maricopa County Medical Society*, 457 U.S. 332.

NASW (National Association of Social Workers), 1997, "Code of Ethics," http://www.naswdc.org/code.htm (1/8/99).

North Carolina, 1991, *General Statutes of North Carolina Chapter 90B: Social Worker Certification Act October 1991,* "Section .0500—Ethical Guidelines," http://www.nccbsw.org/Code.htm (1/8/99).

Orr, Robert D., and Leigh B. Gensen, 1997, "Requests for 'Inappropriate' Treatment Based on Religious Beliefs," *Journal of Medical Ethics*, 23:142–147.

Public Citizen (Health Research Group), 1997, "Hospital Emergency Rooms and Patient Dumping," http://www.citizen.org/hrg/publications/dumping (12/4/99).

Rosenstein, Daniel N., 1993, "Emergency Stabilization for a Wounded COBRA," *Issues in Law and Medicine*, 9(3):255–296.

Shils, Edward B., 1997, "Measuring the Economic and Sociological Impact of the Mega-Retail Discount Chains on Small Enterprise in Urban, Suburban and Rural Communities," http://www.shilsreport.org (5/15/99).

Spielman, Bethany J., 1988, "Financially Motivated Transfers and Discharges: Administrators' Ethics and Public Expectations," *Journal of Medical Humanities and Bioethics*, 9(1):32–43.

Summers, 1996, *Summers v. Baptist Medical Center Arkadelphia*, 69 F3d 902 (8th Circuit) rev on reh 91 F3d 1132 (1996).

Wal-Mart, 1995, *Wal-Mart Stores v. American Drugs Inc.*, 319 Ark. 214, 891 S.W. 2d (Ark 1995).

Wood, Joseph P., 1996, "Emergency Physicians' Obligations to Managed Care Patients under COBRA," *Academic Emergency Medicine*, 3(8):794–800.

Woodstock (Woodstock Theological Center), 1995, *Ethical Considerations in the Business Aspects of Health Care*, Washington, DC: Georgetown University Press.

Yeh, Charlotte, and Nancy Trombly, 1997, "Challenges in the Delivery of ED Care Under COBRA/EMTALA Requirements," http://www.rmf.org/w8458.html (4/19/98).

Zucker, Marjorie B., and Howard D. Zucker, eds., 1997, *Medical Futility and the Evolution of Life-Sustaining Interventions*, Cambridge, UK: Cambridge University Press.

9

COMMUNITY, MEDIA, AND GOVERNMENT RELATIONS

The computer has changed the daily work of public relations professionals as much as it has affected accountants and engineers. Press releases and annual reports may look much the same, but desktop published newsletters and graphics-designed brochures have proliferated, and every organization now needs a Website. The scope of community relations activities has also expanded. Many public relations people run speakers' bureaus, some coordinate volunteer services, and others facilitate self-help groups. Along with the expansion of activities, public relations professionals in healthcare organizations are now expected to assess the social and political environments in which the organization operates for the purpose of guiding activities that affect the community in many ways. Publicity concerning community health programs offered by the organization, for example, has developed into a wide range of networking activities with community organizations to identify needs and implement the delivery of these programs. Healthcare organizations are major property holders, and community relations professionals have found themselves involved in zoning and city planning. Healthcare organizations are major users of public services such as fire and police protection, and public relations professionals may play a role in addressing security problems in their communities. Community relations professionals are now at the forefront of a wide range of organizational activities.

The diversity of community issues is so great and the detail so varied that it is not possible to survey the whole range of these activities. As with the issue of program development in Chapter 6, therefore, I will approach the complex matter of community, media, and government relations by presenting specific cases that illustrate many of the ethical issues involved.

COMMUNITY RELATIONS: THE MEDICAL WASTE INCINERATOR

In the introduction to this book, I mentioned some of the issues associated with the construction of a new medical waste incinerator in my own community in Charleston, West Virginia. My point there was that the issue posed many problems that were beyond the concern of the hospital's clinical ethics committee. The ethics committee heard reports on the issue but did not take up the problem in any active way. Most members of the committee (physicians, nurses, social workers, and clergy) felt that the matter was in the hands of the administrators, and the few who had a specific interest in the problem soon realized that the clinical ethics committee was not the best forum in which to address it. I now want to look at the problem as a case study in organizational ethics and community relations.

Since the late 1980s, the Charleston Area Medical Center (CAMC) had been planning to replace its three medical waste incinerators with one central incinerator. The hospital hired a consultant and did an investigation of alternative processes for medical waste disposal—autoclaving, chemical treatment, and microwaving. It even pilot-tested a chemical/shredding system that did not perform as well as expected. In the early 1990s, CAMC officials decided that the incineration technology would be best and that they should consolidate their waste disposal at the General Division—one of the three campuses into which the hospital is divided. The hospital applied to the West Virginia Health Care Cost Review Authority for a Certificate of Need, a public hearing was held, and the Certificate was issued in 1995. The hospital also needed a city building permit, an air pollution permit from the state Division of Environmental Protection, and a permit for the incinerator from the state Solid Waste Authority.

In 1995, an Air Pollution Permit was issued by the Division of Environmental Protection (DEP). The permit itself proved controversial, however, since it did not set any limits on dioxin emissions. The DEP explained that there were no federal regulations governing dioxin emissions and that the state had no power to set limits. Residents pointed out that the DEP had, in fact, set dioxin emission limits in issuing a permit for a controversial pulp mill a year earlier and that the state agency was empowered to do this. The permit for the paper mill actually said that if the DEP failed to set limits for dioxin emissions, it would be negligent in carrying out its obligations to protect the public health. If dioxin emission limits were needed for the remote area of a pulp mill, the citizens argued, they would surely be needed for a medical waste incinerator in the center of the state's capital city.

Other factual questions were also unanswered. An estimate of dioxin emissions from the planned incinerator prepared by a CAMC engineer stated that the level would be over 50 times the limit set for the pulp mill, although a subsequent report by a CAMC consultant put the estimate well below that limit. The hospital had applied for a permit from the state Solid Waste Authority, and state officials had assured hospital administrators that everything was in order and that the permit would be issued. The city building permit application was also submitted, but this was not considered problematic since it was for the replacement of an existing facility.

In July 1996, CAMC began construction on the new medical waste incinerator at its General Division in the working-class East End of the city. The community response to the announcement that construction had started was immediately negative. There had been no public hearings on permits other than the Health Care Cost Review Authority hearing two years earlier, which was limited to financial considerations; the Authority had no jurisdiction over waste disposal, air pollution, or city planning. Toward the end of July, a public information meeting was held. The meeting was organized by officials from the state Solid Waste Authority and was attended by community relations professionals and other executives from CAMC. Public input was quite emotional and on many points was very well informed. The hospital position was explained, and the CEO promised that CAMC would not operate the incinerator until all problems were resolved.

Shortly after the meeting, residents of the area brought a case in Kanawha County Circuit Court, claiming that all the required permits had not been issued, that the facility would violate state solid waste regulations, and that dangerously high levels of dioxin would be emitted. Kanawha County Circuit Court Judge Robert Smith ruled that the project could go forward, however, since he considered it unlikely that a public hearing would affect the outcome of the permitting process. The issue was unresolved while the remaining permits and the court case were pending. The hospital felt that it had covered all bases and was free to move ahead, while the residents felt that they had been taken by surprise since there had been little publicity and no opportunity for public comment on the environmental issues.

At this point CAMC, through its community relations office, convened an East End Community Roundtable involving about 20 citizens and 5 CAMC administrators. At the first meeting, after many concerns were voiced, it was proposed that a small working group composed of three citizen representatives and three hospital executives meet to consider some of the technical questions. The point of the proposal was to try, first, to agree on the facts since many of the facts themselves were scientifically imprecise or disputed. The working group, chaired by a local businessman who was a member of the CAMC board of trustees, was to report back to the East End Community Roundtable.

As the working group's discussions began, the citizens indicated that the intent of the hospital to burn not only its medical waste but all of its solid waste at the facility was entirely unacceptable. Solid waste incinerators were illegal in the state under a recent law (with the exception of medical waste incinerators), so it would have been illegal even for the city to burn ordinary solid waste. The possibility did exist that all CAMC solid waste could be designated medical waste and incinerated. This would have been challenged legally and, in any case, was clearly against the spirit of the law. The CAMC officials agreed.

The issue of dioxin emissions focused the attention of the working group on the problems of separating medical waste from other solid waste, including or excluding dioxin-producing plastics, and the hospital's method of dealing with its waste stream. Additional professional advice was needed, and a new consultant (one proposed by the citizens and acceptable to the hospital) was hired to analyze the waste stream itself and to develop a new plan. On the basis of new information, CAMC reevaluated its cost/benefit estimates for the project and essentially agreed with the position taken by the community representatives. The community representatives accepted the fact that, given present technology, incineration of toxic medical waste was the best alternative.

Ultimately, the small working group developed a mutually acceptable solution to the whole problem and did not bring it back to the East End Roundtable. The Charleston Area Medical Center agreed to run the incinerator at less than a quarter of the capacity originally proposed, to burn only toxic medical waste, to exclude as much dioxin-producing plastic as possible from the medical waste, to redesign its waste disposal system on the basis of a new waste stream analysis, to maintain citizen review of the operation of the incinerator, and to continue to elicit citizen input on a whole range of community concerns. The citizens agreed to accept the incineration of toxic medical waste on this basis and to cooperate with the project. The citizen lawsuit was withdrawn, and a formal agreement was signed.

The solution of this problem was a remarkable exercise in community relations. Although discussions began with resentment on both sides, an atmosphere of cooperation and trust eventually developed in the working group. Good will and flexibility are essential to any process like this. If the people involved had been more concerned with building their own professional careers or their positions of influence in the community through accusations and stonewalling, the process would not have been successful.

In this case, two factors helped immensely. First, the citizens involved were not only community leaders trusted by their neighbors, but they were willing to invest time and energy to become fully conversant with the many political, legal, economic, and technical aspects of the issue. The knowledge and common sense of the citizen participants gained the respect of the hospital administrators. Second, on the part of the hospital, the single most important element was the fact that the CEO became an active member of the working group. The community representatives thus knew that they were talking with the key decision makers. The group would have been imbalanced if the hospital representatives had to report to higher-level administrators at each step and the administrators making the decisions were a stage removed from citizen interaction. The involvement of the CEO increased the flexibility of the hospital in its consideration of alternatives and signified to the citizens that the institution was serious in its negotiations.

There were strong social and economic pressures on both sides. The community representatives were politically accountable to a very diverse group of citizens, some of whom would settle for nothing less than the elimination of the incinerator. There were many citizen organizations with different leaders and different interests: the *public* is not a homogeneous group. On the hospital side, there were various safety and engineering administrators who did not want to appear to have been wrong about earlier decisions and, of course, CAMC had already invested considerable resources in the project. A long and very public court battle would have cost the hospital a great deal of time and money, not to mention the serious loss of community good will.

In terms of the ethics of community relations, the lessons to be learned from this case are important. First, institutions should take public sentiment seriously, even when concern does not arise spontaneously. It cannot be assumed that there is no public interest just because complaints have not been formally submitted. This requires active listening on the part of community relations professionals and the development of a corporate posture that treats the community as a partner—a genuine stakeholder. Second, early warning signs need to be heeded; if public objections reach a state of outrage, as was almost the case with the CAMC incinerator, it may be too late. Third, an orderly process of dealing with the public is essential. The public may well act inconsistently, but the organization cannot afford to do so. The quest for order, however, must not lead to an institutional approach that simply develops a plan and then tries to sell it to the public. If they are to be real stakeholders, community members need to be involved in every stage of the process and empowered to participate meaningfully. This is what is necessary if one is to take seriously the public mission of an organization and the interests of its community stakeholders.

In the jargon of business management, community relations professionals are sometimes referred to as *boundary spanners* who represent the corporation to the public, on the one hand, and the public to the corporation, on the other. They must act in the interests of the company, according to Donna J. Wood, but they also have a responsibility to represent public interests fairly to people inside the organization.

Sometimes they must convince company insiders that external interests should take precedence over what the firm defines as its own interests. . . . The boundary-spanner's position is thus politically difficult, which makes it all the more important that the function have credibility and status within the organization.

(Wood, 1990:511)

The task of presenting community perspectives to chief operating officers and boards of directors can be as difficult as the task of representing the organization to the public. Often governing boards and chief executives want only a press officer, who will stage public events to get free media coverage, or an information office that will publish materials presenting the corporation in the best light. These high-level decision makers do not always want to hear what the public really thinks—or they prefer to believe that their own conceptions of public opinion are accurate. Representing the public to the organization faithfully is in many respects the crucial ethical dimension of the boundary spanner's responsibility. It requires a degree of advocacy on behalf of the public stakeholders and, at times, an appeal to the collective conscience of the organization to remember its own mission.

There is, therefore, a professional obligation involved in the work of community relations officers. The community relations professional has an ethical obligation to present the facts honestly, much as lawyers, accountants, physicians, and nurses have ethical obligations to their professions. This obligation is both a source of strength, since ultimate decision makers need to know the social and political consequences of their decisions, and a responsibility to the organization's outside stakeholders. Community relations professionals can play a larger role in developing the ethical dimension of organizational activities than was the case in the past (Fitzpatrick, 1996).

Organizational mission statements often mention responsibilities to the community. The Mission of Satilla Regional Medical Center, for example, states that one of its goals is "to care for and improve the quality of life of our community" (Satilla, 1997). With or without such explicit recognition, it must be acknowledged that the community served by a healthcare organization is a primary stakeholder in its operations. Physicians and nurses may meet the healthcare needs of individual patients, but from a sociological perspective, the organization itself is directed to the collective healthcare needs of the community. The business decisions of the healthcare organization are at issue here, as well as its patient care and public education programs.

Case 9.1 The Hospital That Ruined the Neighborhood

Seneca Community Hospital had grown too big for its neighborhood. It was founded in the mid-1970s when the then rural area was developing into a suburb. The hospital was only 20 miles from a hospital three times its size, but it became a major healthcare provider in its own right. It had an association with the medical school at the state university through which it had residency programs in family practice, internal medicine, and pediatrics. A long-term care facility built in 1995 added 60 beds to its 220 acute care beds. The hospital's location between the town center and the interstate highway was not ideal. Unfortunately, it was not on the main road, but three blocks off the highway in the middle of a residential neighborhood.

In an attempt to solve a growing problem with parking, the hospital purchased 2.7 acres to the west of its medical office building. This was the only available land that was adjacent to hospital property since it had purchased land to the east in 1989 for its outpatient and emergency department expansion. The prospect of a new parking building, however, was upsetting many people in the immediate neighborhood. There had been grumbling for some time about the increased traffic on the residential streets. The hospital had placed signs on the main road directing patients and visitors to use one entrance, medical office building patients to use another street, and nursing home traffic to use yet another approach. The traffic was making the neighborhood unsafe. Ambulance drivers were aware of the problem of driving through residential neighborhoods, but the people following the ambulances or arriving on their own in emergency situations posed a real hazard.

The hospital's parking problem involved a conflict of rights and interests between people in the immediate neighborhood and the wider community served by the hospital. The conflicting interests were clear, and no solution was acceptable to all. One ethical concern was the question of how far the hospital should go to involve community leaders in the search for a solution. Would it have been better to involve them from the outset in considering whatever options might be available, or to come up with a plan to present to the community with the hope of having it accepted? While it may be tempting to formulate a plan first, a hospital that treats its community as a real stakeholder would find a number of advantages in involving community leaders early in the process. As things turned out, the plan that the hospital presented to the community was scrapped after a brief but heated meeting, and an alternative involving parking restrictions and one-way streets was adopted.

MEDIA RELATIONS

Media relations can present some very difficult problems. Corporations, like individuals, have tentative positions and plans that they are not ready to reveal to the public. Premature disclosure of incomplete plans can jeopardize business deals and create needless public alarm that may be difficult to dispel later. One is always suspicious of secrecy, however—especially on the part of organizations that have public responsibilities. The public does have a right to know, and delay in disclosing the details may prevent people from taking actions they would want to take. Many of the most difficult media problems thus have to do with the timing of the release of information rather than with the ultimate disclosure of facts.

Again, let me use a case presentation to address this issue, recognizing that this can present only some of the many issues involved. This case involves a managed care program, Carelink Health Plans, a joint venture of Camcare, Inc., a nonprofit corporation, and Charleston Health Associates, a West Virginia physicians' association. Carelink began operations in 1994 as an MCO, with a $30 million investment from its parent corporation. The field was wide open: only 4% of the state's health-insured population was covered by managed care in 1995. By 1997 Carelink had enrolled over 60,000 members from over 400 employer groups, the Public Employees Insurance Agency, Medicare, and Medicaid. Its provider network included more than 1300 participating physicians and 29 hospitals. Revenues grew from $26 million in 1996 to $78 million in 1997. The plan was accredited by the NCQA in 1997. It stated its corporate philosophy briefly as follows:

> To meet the needs of the customers, providers and owners we serve, Carelink will operate an accountable managed care system for the improvement of health, emphasizing choice and compassion in the provision of health care services.
>
> (Camcare, 1998)

Although Carelink was the largest MCO in the state by 1998, it had not yet turned the corner financially and was still operating at more of a loss than had been expected. The operating loss of $7.8 million in 1997 was down slightly from $8.0 million in 1996, but not nearly enough to attain profitability within five years, as anticipated. While this was a serious crisis for Carelink, it was not uncommon, given the financial conditions that every managed care program faces in its early phases. For a certain number of start-up years, any managed care plan is expected to operate at a loss. By 1997 MCO enrollment was up to 11% of the state population, but five of the seven plans in the state were still operating at a loss. State and industry officials questioned whether West Virginia, with its small population and the problems of health care delivery in rural areas, could sustain seven MCOs. Carelink was competitive, however, having gained 29% of the enrollees in the market area.

Plan administrators attributed losses to higher than predicted medical costs (Carelink, 1998). At 94.1% of revenues, however, Carelink medical payments were about average for plans operating in the state. West Virginia is not a healthy state—it ranks first in heart disease, third in diabetes and cancer, and fourth in tobacco use. It also has the highest median age of any state. Administrative expenses at 15.5% of revenue were close to target levels for this stage of Carelink's development but were still higher than those of other plans in the state (some were as low as 8%) and much higher than could be sustained for a population with such high medical costs.

In May 1998, Carelink received an annual report from its external auditor, Arthur Anderson, that posed a number of public relations problems. The cover letter to the report contained the usual statements concerning generally accepted auditing standards and assurances that the Carelink financial statements constituted a fair representation of the company's financial condition. The cover letter also included the following qualifications:

> The accompanying financial statements have been prepared assuming that the Company will continue as a going concern. As discussed in Note 1 to the financial statements, the Company has suffered recurring losses from operations and has a net capital deficiency that raises substantial doubt about its ability to continue as a going concern.

Note 1 read, in part:

> The Company's operating losses were due primarily to higher than expected physician and pharmacy health care costs. The Company has borrowed $7,320,000 in 1997 and $6,700,000 in 1996 from Camcare to sustain its working capital needs and to meet the minimum statutory reserve requirements. Management is budgeting a loss of approximately $6,600,000 for 1998.
>
> Management has enacted a number of strategic initiatives for 1998 to reduce the Company's budgeted loss. These strategic initiatives include renegotiating physician contracts, improving the COB and subrogation recovery process, and implementing additional utilization, disease and case management programs. There are no assurances that these plans will be successful or that the Company will be able to obtain additional borrowings or capital.
>
> (Carelink, 1998:16,21)

Carelink was required to send the Audit Report and notes to the state Insurance Commission, and it would then become public.

The Carelink response to the Audit Report and any possible action by the state Insurance Commission was important. Loss of public confidence in the plan could keep enrollments from reaching the projected breakeven level. Losses per member per month had dropped from $41 in 1996 to $9 in 1997, and maintaining enrollment was essential. One MCO operating in the state had experienced a loss of membership the previous year after raising its prices. Physician confidence and cooperation was another issue. While many physicians in the Carelink service area had joined the plan, others had refused. Some physicians undoubtedly felt that they had little or no choice but to join, some found the terms of the contract unacceptable, and some felt that the plan had treated them poorly. Carelink's relationship to its parent, Camcare, was also strained. While Camcare and Carelink had worked very closely, the Camcare board of directors had to reevaluate its own commitment to its subsidiary in light of the prevailing financial situation, and this meant that any publicity surrounding the Audit Report would have an effect on the local and state financial community.

The financial crisis faced by Carelink is not our concern, but rather the decision making involved in its relations with the media. Camcare/Carelink public relations officers faced a number of questions:

1. Would it be appropriate for the public relations office to delay making the Audit Report public while Carelink developed an appropriate response?
2. Should preparing a public response include prior discussion with the Insurance Commissioner?
3. The effect of the Audit Report and the subsequent publicity might not be entirely negative. The Audit Report itself notified physicians that the operating losses were due in large part to high physician and pharmacy costs. An organizational response emphasizing this might place Carelink in a better position to renegotiate physician contracts and fee schedules, but if the plan placed too much blame on the physicians, it could undermine those important relationships. How should this be managed?
4. All things considered, how should a response be formulated that would be fair to all stakeholders and reflect Carelink's mission?

As things turned out, there was little opportunity for delay. The press was alert and picked up the Audit Report as soon as it was forwarded to the Insurance Commission. Camcare President and CEO Phillip Goodwin and Insurance Commissioner Hanley Clark spoke to a reporter from the *Charleston Daily Mail*. The Camcare/Carelink public relations staff formulated a response that included information about the development of Carelink health and prevention programs, customer satisfaction reports, graphs showing the drastic reduction in operating expenses, comparisons of incomes and losses with those of other plans, and a covering letter from Alan L. Mytty, president and CEO of Carelink. According to Mytty:

> Carelink managers are taking steps to eliminate losses so that break-even will occur in 1999, our fifth year of operation. Major initiatives include new physician fee schedules, more efficient administrative services, computer system enhancements, rate adjustments and more effective utilization management.
>
> (Carelink, 1998:3)

The Insurance Commission announced an investigation into Carelink's financial problems, but the comments of the Insurance Commissioner reported in the paper were generally supportive of the Plan.

> "The financial status they find themselves in is not unusual," Clark said of Carelink. "It takes time for an HMO to understand the medical and financial circumstances of their clientele. This is not something for the public to be concerned with. . . . Our role is to stay on top and work with HMOs," Clark said. "The public should watch the financial status of HMOs, but they have no reason to feel any of ours will become insolvent."
>
> (Cox, 1998:1A)

Ethically, there were a number of stakeholder interests to be considered. Potential consumers had a right to know whatever information they considered to be relevant to their choice of entering, leaving, or remaining in the plan. Plan members had an interest in the solvency of the plan—an interest that coincided with the responsibility of the Insurance Commissioner. Camcare had an interest in its investment. Physicians had an interest in judging the financial stability of the plan if they were to enter into contractual relations with it. And, of course, Carelink administrators and employees had an interest in the plan's success.

The public relations question was how to be fair to each group in presenting information to the public. Presenting the organization in the best possible light is, of course, the major responsibility of the public relations professional. This duty must be balanced, however, by the duty to treat all parties fairly. It is quite clear to public relations professionals today that misrepresentations, cover-ups, glosses, withholding relevant information, and distorting "spin" are likely to be counterproductive. These practices undermine the credibility of the public relations office with the media and reduce the trust of the organization's stakeholders.

This much having been said, the devil is still in the details. The daily life of media representatives and publications professionals is still a matter of presenting the organization in the best possible light. What an ethical perspective can contribute to the task is the guidance that can be drawn from a strong appreciation of the mission of the institution and its responsibility to its stakeholders. It cannot lay out a cookbook approach of guidelines that will apply to all situations, but it can provide principles to be considered at those times when the pressure is strong.

GOVERNMENT RELATIONS

The fastest-growing and most rapidly changing areas of organizational activity are perhaps the most dangerous from an ethical perspective. With the exception of computer technology, health care has been the fastest-growing and most rapidly changing sector of the American economy since the 1960s. As a percentage of the gross domestic product, health care expanded from 5.3% in 1960 to 14.2% in 1993, with an average annual cost per capita rising from $143 in 1964 to $3380 in 1993 (HCFA, 1993). There are fortunes to be made in health care, power bases to be established, careers to be launched, markets to be cornered, and often temptations to be resisted.

The cutting edge of this economic development has been governmental relations. The boom of the last 30 years originated with the establishment of the Medicare program in the early 1960s and was drastically curtailed with the development of the federal prospective payment system in the 1980s. Through Medicare, Medicaid, the Veterans Administration, the National Institutes of Health, and many other major programs, federal and state governments now finance over 40% of American hospital care. With the introduction of managed care in the 1990s, and the prospect of further federal and state control of health plans to protect patient rights, the rules of the game have changed again. Government regulations have had a pervasive influence on healthcare organizations. As a result, lobbying ("the process of influencing public officials to promote or secure the passage or defeat of legislation" [Carroll, 1993]) and government relations (working with government agency officials to influence the regulation and administration of programs) have become crucial activities for healthcare organizations.

Contrary to its popular image, lobbying plays an important role in government. Lobbyists bring to government a wealth of information and experience that public officials otherwise would not have. Legislators and public officials have staff to collect and sort through information, but these people have only limited access to crucial information and often lack the experience necessary for the task. While the product of our political process is not always the best, the opportunity for both sides to have a hearing generally exists, and there is always another round to be fought since legislation can be amended at any time.

This does not mean, however, that current lobbying practices are acceptable. By common consensus, "big money" plays too large a political role in the United States. From both public interest and industry perspectives, lobbying tactics and the influence of political campaign contributions need to be brought under control. Efforts to wield political influence are no more beneficial to healthcare organizations than to the public interest. In the first place, it can be expensive, drawing off funds that could be used to further the basic service objectives of the organization. Second, it can bring negative publicity. Finally, and most important, the mission of a healthcare organization can be lost in the fray. As political battles escalate and the costs of campaign contributions get higher, the public interest is neglected and the less powerful (employees, the uninsured, and the elderly) tend to lose out. One cannot fault individuals or organizations that attempt to work within the current system: advocacy is both legitimate and important to the political process. But it is not inconsistent for an organization to play by the current rules and, at the same time, to advocate changing the rules to improve the game. While they devote resources to policy research and government relations, therefore, healthcare organizations also have a deep interest in bringing the system under control.

Repealing the Transfer Provision

The important difference between a narrow focus on financial benefit to organizations and a broader concern for the public good is evident in one item on the AHA's advocacy agenda for 1998 (AHA, 1998a, 1998b). The Balanced

Budget Act of 1997 applied new reimbursement rules to ten Medicare DRG payment categories. Previously, when patients were transferred from one hospital to another, payments would be divided proportionately between the two facilities. When patients were discharged to nursing facilities, rehabilitation services, or home health care, however, the hospital would receive full payment according to the DRG schedule. Even if the hospital stay had been shorter than anticipated, Medicare would begin paying for nursing facility, rehabilitation, or home health services, while it still paid the full amount to the hospital. Congress felt that Medicare was paying double for these days and reclassified the transition to these other services as transfers rather than discharges so that payments to the hospitals would be cut off when the payments to the other services began.

The AHA, however, pointed out that the Medicare prospective payment system was originally established to offer hospitals a financial incentive for efficiency (AHA, 1998c). An average length of stay was built into the payment calculation for each DRG, knowing that in some cases patients would stay longer and in others they would be discharged sooner. The idea behind the system was to reward hospitals for reducing the length of stay. But now, if hospitals no longer were paid the full amount for patients who could leave early, two things would happen. First, hospitals would not have the funds from the early discharges to cover the costs of those patients who had to stay beyond the projected time for the DRG; second, hospitals might keep patients for the full length of stay in order to collect full payment. So while it may seem reasonable for Medicare to want to reduce payments for discharges to other services by reclassifying them as transfers, this would really remove the incentives that were originally built into the DRG system itself and, according to the AHA, penalize those hospitals that should be rewarded. The AHA makes an important point here: Congress should have considered the effects of its cost-cutting action on the incentives involved in the prospective payment system.

There are points to be made on either side of this issue: taxpayers should not have to pay double for early transfers, but this is a significant part of the economic incentive built into the Medicare system. In addition to the economic issue, however, this conflict raises the ethical question of the public duty of healthcare providers. Should hospitals and their advocacy associations such as the AHA act solely to promote the financial interests of the industry, or do they have a public responsibility to develop an efficient healthcare system? By supporting a bill to repeal the transfer provision, the AHA is advocating a position that would benefit its members. It would not solve the problem of the double payments under the previous federal rules. Does a hospital have any reason to be concerned about the cost to the public under different sets of regulations? If the healthcare organization's mission involves responsibility to society, or if the government and ultimately the taxpayers are considered stakeholders in the system of which the healthcare organization is a part, one might expect hospitals to accept some responsibility for helping to find a fair solution to the problem rather than just adopting a position that serves their own financial interests. Repeal of the transfer provision is not enough. If the AHA's analysis of the likely effects of the provisions of the 1997 Balanced Budget Act is correct, an alternative solution is needed—one that reflects a more public responsibility.

CONCLUSIONS

The extent to which a healthcare organization sees itself not only as providing healthcare services to individuals, but also as an organization dedicated to improving the community, should be reflected in its mission statement. The community has a stake in how the healthcare organization conducts its business—a stake that comes to the fore whenever organizational actions affect community interests. These interests involve environmental issues, public safety, zoning, employment, and other community concerns in addition to health services. Community relations involve public interests as well as organizational objectives, and healthcare organizations must respect the responsibility of community relations professionals to find an appropriate balance among the many values involved. Media relations directly reflect the attitude of an organization toward its community and play an important role in establishing the trust that is essential to a cooperative relationship. Government relations should be conducted with a sense of the greater public interest in mind, not just the immediate interests of the organization. The organizational code of conduct should contain standards requiring those who represent the institution to be fair and honest in their community, media, and governmental relations.

REFERENCES

AHA (American Hospital Association), 1998a, "False Claims Act and Medicare Billing Disputes," http://www.aha.org/grassroots/medbillerrorsL1.html (6/6/98).
——, 1998b, "Bill Summary H.R. 3523: The Health Care Claims Guidance Act of 1998," http://www.aha.org/grassroots/medbillerrorsL1.html (6/7/98).
——, 1998c, "Advocacy Papers from the 1998 Annual Meeting," http://www.aha.org/repeal.html (6/7/98).
Camcare, 1998, "Camcare Health System," http://www.camcare.com/sitemenu.html (8/25/98).
Carelink, 1998, "Progress Report and Audited Statement," Charleston, WV: Carelink Health Plans, Inc.
Carroll, Archie B., 1993, *Business and Society: Ethics and Stakeholder Management*, 2nd ed., Cincinnati: South-Western Publishing Company.
Cox, Theresa, 1998, "Carelink Losses Probed," *Charleston Daily Mail*, July 24,:1A.

Fitzpatrick, Kathy R., 1996, "The Role of Public Relations in the Institutionalization of Ethics," *Public Relations Review*, 22(3):249–258.

HCFA (Health Care Financing Administration), 1993, "HCFA Statistics," Pub. No. 03341, Washington, DC: U.S. Department of Health and Human Services.

Satilla (Satilla Regional Medical Center, Waycross, GA), 1997, "Vision and Mission Statement," http://www.satilla.org/ (1/12/99).

Wood, Donna J., 1990, *Business and Society*, New York: HarperCollins Publishers.

10

EMPLOYEE RELATIONS

Employment opportunities in the hospital sector increased in the 1990s: by 2.7% for full-time employees and 5.2% for part-time employees between 1992 and 1996 (AHA, 1998). This does not mean that employees' jobs are secure, however. The rise in outpatient services and home health care during this period must be considered in light of layoffs due to the decline in inpatient utilization. While registered nurse employment increased over this period, licensed practical nurse employment decreased. Recent cuts in federal programs, furthermore, may lead to continued downsizing of staff in certain sectors. In health care, as in other sectors of the economy, employees are nervous about job security (Caudron, 1996).

The shift of power from hospitals to managed care plans and insurance companies has exacerbated the problem. Middle-level administrators fear that they may be laid off, and direct care givers worry that they will be short-staffed and overloaded with duties beyond their professional capabilities. Reorganization often moves administrative decision making further away from caregivers and imposes a less personal regime on employees. The more distant management becomes, the more employees feel that decisions are made on the basis of some hidden agenda or that the administration's agenda is no longer in touch with the daily problems of direct care. All of this results in considerable stress on employee relations.

This chapter explores the ethical dimension of employee relations in health-care organizations. It begins with an analysis of the ethical basis of employment and moves on to specific problems in the areas of hiring, evaluation, promotion, and dismissal. It addresses employees' right to privacy, whistle-blowing, and union organization and concludes with some brief comments on occupational health and safety.

ETHICAL PERSPECTIVES

The ethical obligations of employers to employees, and vice versa, are not well established. In the last part of the nineteenth century, the doctrine of *employment at will* became legally recognized in the United States. This doctrine holds that if there is no specific contract between the employer and the employee, an employee can be legally dismissed for no reason at all or even (as the Tennessee Supreme Court once said) for a reason that is morally wrong (Paine, 1884). The doctrine gave rise to abusive conditions for workers, who had little choice but to accept them. In 1897 New York State passed a law limiting the hours bakers could work to ten per day, six days a week. This law was ruled unconstitutional by the U.S. Supreme Court on the grounds that it interfered with the Fourteenth Amendment right of the bakers and the bakery owners to enter into contracts by depriving them of liberty and property without due process (Lochner, 1905).

Only since the 1930s have serious legal restrictions been placed on the freedom of employers to set the terms and conditions of employment. Laws limiting hours and fixing minimum wages were enacted, along with laws regulating benefits and giving employees the right to organize labor unions and engage in collective bargaining. Civil rights laws passed in the 1960s and later gave equal opportunity to job applicants of all races and both sexes and protected workers from discrimination. Major health and safety regulations were passed in the 1970s. Beyond these laws, however, employees still have only the rights specified in their employment agreements.

Apart from these rather limited restraints, the treatment of employees ultimately depends on the ethical perspective of the employer. Employers can recognize employees' claims to fair hiring, reasonable evaluation, opportunity for advancement, equitable pay, favorable working conditions, effective hearing of grievances, respect for privacy, and security from unjust or sudden termination if they wish, or they can refuse to acknowledge these rights. Employment contracts, whether with unions or with individual employees, are merely ways of specifying these conditions of employment.

What, then, is the ethical basis of employer–employee relations? In general, there have been two approaches to this question. The first is a defense of the employment at will doctrine; the second is based on claims to a more extensive set of workers' rights. The former (traditionally an employers' perspective) has been used to limit workers' rights, the latter (a workers' perspective) to expand them.

Employment at Will

The doctrine of employment at will has been defended in two ways. First, it is justified on the basis of the liberty and property rights that can be claimed as natural human rights protected by the U.S. Constitution. From this perspective, the right to enter into an employment contract is comparable to the right to free speech, trial by jury, or religious belief (Epstein, 1984). If liberty and the ownership of property (i.e., property used in business) are human rights, according to this defense, the government has no right to interfere with employment contracts.

This defense of employment at will is ethically naive. The equality of power presupposed by the concept of a free contract simply does not exist (Velasquez, 1998:462). If one shifts the focus of this concept from a narrow concern for the contractual relationship to the consequences of the doctrine, it becomes clear that without certain protections, such as due process with regard to dismissal, a minimum wage, and occupational safety regulations, free employment contracts are morally unacceptable because they give employers control over the lives of workers (Scanlon, 1977). The great majority of the labor force is simply not free to do without employment or to change working conditions they cannot accept.

Employment at will has also been defended on utilitarian grounds. Freedom of contract, according to this perspective, works to the advantage of both employers and employees (Epstein, 1984). If employees do not view an at-will contract as beneficial in light of the alternatives, they simply will not accept it. This theory is often supported by claims to the effect that employees can control working conditions by threatening to quit, so they actually have more power than if they were under a contract for employment for a fixed term.

The utilitarian analysis, however, is no more persuasive than the liberty defense. To argue that employees will not accept a contract that is not to their advantage begs the question. It assumes that employees are free to choose from among a set of alternatives when in fact the company is not offering any alternatives. What is offered is either at-will employment or no work at all. Employees do not normally have the option of seeking a better contract at another company. Only if the at-will contract were offered as an alternative to other choices such as contracts with due process, fair wages, and occupational safety could the utilitarian value to the worker be judged acceptable. For utilitarian maximization to justify a choice, alternatives must be considered.

Arguments against employment at will have focused almost exclusively on employee protection against unjust dismissal (Boatright, 1997). This has done great disservice to the ethical evaluation of employee relations because it has left all other employee concerns out of the equation. When the focus of the debate is simply the acceptance or rejection of employment and all other aspects of employment are subsumed under the notion of contractual acceptance or rejection, employee relations are not adequately addressed. Important as it has been historically, the employment at will doctrine is socially naive and much too narrow to serve as an ethical framework for employee relations.

Employee Rights

The second ethical approach to employee relations addresses not only the freedom to accept or reject employment, but the whole range of employment. It is often claimed that employees have certain rights in the workplace based on their natural rights as persons and their civil rights as granted by society. Typically employees' rights include due process with regard to employment decisions, protection from discrimination, collective bargaining, fair compensation, whistle-blowing, personal privacy, and occupational health and safety. Employee obligations include loyalty to the interests of the organization, protection of proprietary information, respect for organizational property, and acceptable work performance (De George, 1990; Werhane, 1985).

Employee rights can be defended on utilitarian grounds as beneficial to workers, employers, and society at large in the long run, but the more common ethical justification flows from the concept of human integrity. Respect for the integrity of individuals as a basic ethical principle is thought to require the acknowledgment of employee rights in the workplace (De George, 1990). Basic human rights were traditionally considered to have either a rational justification (individuals want their own integrity respected and therefore must respect the integrity of others) or a natural justification (certain rights are necessary to a fully human life). More recently, a contractual justification (people in an ideal society would agree to establish civil rights) has been more influential. These justifications are often supported by the claim that society has historically recognized human rights. In addition to upholding constitutional and statutory rights in the United States (free speech, civil rights, occupational safety, a minimum wage, etc.), defenders of this moral justification also point to the Universal Declaration of Human Rights of the United Nations. The Declaration begins with the claim that "recognition of the inherent dignity and of the equal and inalienable rights of all members of the human family is the foundation of freedom, justice and peace in the world" (UN, 1948). It elaborates specific employment rights as "the right to work, to free choice of employment, to just and favorable conditions of work and to protection against unemployment . . .

the right to equal pay for equal work . . . the right to just and favorable remu-neration . . . the right to form and to join trade unions . . . [and] the right to rest and leisure, including reasonable limitation of working hours and periodic holidays with pay." While the Universal Declaration of Human Rights may arguably be considered an international policy, it does not have the force of law in sovereign states. Only certain employee rights are established in law and public policy in the United States, so principles such as fair compensation and due process in decisions with regard to hiring, promotion, discipline, and dis-missal remain matters of ethical commitment for the organizations involved.

Stakeholders and Organizational Goals

Stakeholder and organizational goals perspectives shed a slightly different light on the ethics of employee relations. When employees are said to be key stake-holders in a healthcare organization, however, it is not simply because they are viewed as important assets. The stakeholder perspective conceives of employee welfare as one of the aims of the organization itself. Employees are important not only for what they can do *for* the organization, but also because they are primary stakeholders *of* the organization. Employees, along with other stake-holders, are principals. Few people have more at stake in the organization's operations than its employees; organizational decisions affect their lives and livelihood.

Healthcare organizational mission statements often mention employees, fre-quently as an asset to the organization but also as partners or stakeholders. Some mention a commitment to fair employment practices and to equal oppor-tunity, regardless of gender, race, ethnicity, or religion. The most effective mis-sion statements, however, specify appropriate employment and employee wel-fare as organizational goals. Community Hospital in Columbus, Ohio, for example, promises not only a high level of service, but also "an atmosphere conducive to employee empowerment and teamwork" (Columbus, 1998). From the perspectives adopted here, therefore, healthcare organizations should look beyond the concepts of fair employment contracts and employee rights in the workplace when setting their goals. They should recognize employees as key stakeholders in the organization and adopt goals that publicly commit the orga-nization to their welfare and human development.

A final ethical aspect of employee relations involves the role of the profes-sional human resource manager. While all administrators deal with employee relations to the extent that they have supervisory responsibilities, human re-source managers play a unique role. Professional human resource management standards establish a dual set of obligations: responsibilities to the organization and its mission on the one hand, and direct obligations to employees on the other. The first Code of Ethics of the American Society for Personnel Administration (now the Society for Human Resource Management) contained the following provisions:

> Each Member of the American Society for Personnel Administration shall:
> . . . Help create an environment of recognition and support of human values in the workplace.
> . . . Display a unity of spirit and cohesiveness of purpose in bringing fair and equitable treatment of all people to the forefront of employers' thought.
> . . . Provide employees and the public with a sense of confidence about the conduct and intentions of management.
>
> (Chruden and Sherman, 1984:18)

The language of this code may now seem a little dated, but it contains two points not always found in later formulations: (1) the idea that human resource administrators have a duty to bring equitable treatment of employees to "the forefront of employers' thought" and (2) the notion that an emphasis on human values implies employee confidence in the "intentions of management." In many respects, the most important outcome of an ethical approach to employee relations is to ensure that the welfare of employees is regularly addressed at the highest levels of organizational decision making. All too often, decisions concerning financial matters, corporate strategy, and program development are made with the assumption that bringing the workforce into line is simply a managerial function that human resource professionals can handle. This assumption is inadequate, however, when the organizational mission statement acknowledges a serious commitment to employees. The human resource administrator has a specific professional obligation to maintain trust throughout the workforce by representing the interests of employees in organizational decision making.

EMPLOYMENT PRACTICES

The ethical dimension of employment practices can be conceived as a matter of fundamental fairness. Organizations are looking for the best employees they can find, and employees are looking for fair treatment, adequate compensation, advancement opportunities, and fulfilling employment. It is when ambitions override the sense of fairness that problems develop, that is, when organizations attempt to squeeze too much productivity out of too few employees or when employees expect greater compensation than their contribution is worth. The sense of fairness required here, however, must include the notion that labor is not just one factor in the economics of production (De George, 1990; Joseph F. Fletcher, 1960, personal communication).

Hiring

Fundamental fairness in employee selection is not at all inconsistent with organizational efficiency. The best way for organizations to obtain the most talented employees is to use the most effective methods of applicant evaluation; and these, in turn, are the methods that give every qualified applicant an equal opportunity. The most important part of any selection process is to adapt the criteria to the requirements of the positions. Human resource management professionals (including industrial psychologists and industrial relations engineers) have devoted a great deal of research to employee selection (Milkovich and Boudreau, 1988). The basic consideration is whether selection criteria are valid. The evaluation process can be considered valid to the extent that it either (*1*) predicts success on the job or (*2*) measures knowledge, skills, or abilities that are genuinely relevant to the position.

The strongest indication of the validity of selection criteria is a high correlation between test scores and interview ratings at the time of application and subsequent job performance. This determination can involve a complicated procedure for an organization. Although in many cases the evidence (application test scores and subsequent employee evaluations) already exists, it is seldom used to judge the validity of preemployment screening. Evidence of the validity of selection procedures from within the organization can be especially useful if hiring practices are questioned by workers or challenged by applicants. The best defense against charges of favoritism or discrimination is a clear demonstration that the system is fair because there is a direct correlation between selection criteria and job performance.

The alternative approach to employee selection criteria is the evaluation of applicants on the basis of job descriptions. The important point here is that the skills and abilities evaluated (whether by tests, interviews, or employment records) must be relevant to the positions for which employees are being selected. This relevance, in turn, can be assured by comparing the skills and abilities evaluated with the requirements listed in job descriptions. A test of general mathematical or reading abilities for a position in which these abilities play only a very small part would not be a valid use of applicant testing. Testing covers a wide range of skills and abilities, but it is no more effective or fair to applicants than the relevance of the abilities tested to the actual job requirements.

Applicant testing has been criticized and legally challenged in recent years. There was considerable merit to claims made in the 1980s that intelligence tests favored white, middle-class applicants because the content was closer to their backgrounds than to those of minorities. Students of the social sciences are generally aware of the requirements of validity (whether the test measures what it is intended to measure) and reliability (consistency) for testing. The added factor for employee selection is legitimacy: whether the abilities, skills, or knowledge measured are relevant to the requirements of the position. Tests of characteristics unrelated to job specifications can be discriminatory and can eliminate potentially valuable employees from consideration. The criterion of legitimacy was addressed in the U.S. Supreme Court case of *Griggs v. Duke Power Company* (1971), where the Court found it discriminatory for a company to require a high school education and a certain score on a general intelligence test without evidence that these requirements were at all related to job performance.

Applicant testing is not the only form of employee selection, nor is it the most widely used. Applicants are also commonly judged on the basis of biographical information, education, experience, references, and interviews. Legitimacy is still the relevant criterion, however, so these procedures need to be evaluated in relation to their prediction of job performance and actual job requirements. It is no more fair or efficient for an interview or a background check to focus on irrelevant items than for a test to measure skills unrelated to the job. All too often, however, interviews are conducted, references are read, or education is evaluated with little or no comparison to the actual requirements of the position for which the applicants are being evaluated. Oddly enough, the higher in the organization one goes, the less likely it is that actual job requirements will be considered in detail and the more likely it is that decisions will depend solely on the candidate's reputation and personal demeanor. Interviewing applicants always presents the danger that stereotypes may be unconsciously invoked. Human resource specialists have developed ways of compensating for unintended bias, especially through the use of structured interviews (Dessler, 1997:217–245), but it is important that these techniques be kept current.

Studies of the comparative value of various methods of selecting employees from among a group of applicants have found that tests of ability, biographical inventories, records of work experience, and reference checks rate higher than education and training as predictors of future performance (Hunter and Hunter, 1984). Unstructured interviews and quick reference checks, however, are the selection methods most often used (BNA, 1983). According to a report from the Bureau of National Affairs, "An American Management Association survey of over 1,000 employers showed a decline in 1998 in the percentage of employers that test job applicants for basic skills" (BNA, 1998). Many organizations apparently could do more to make hiring both fair to candidates and effective for the organization.

It should also be noted that the Americans with Disabilities Act (ADA) generally prohibits the use of medical information in making employment decisions except where it relates to bona fide occupational qualifications. Medical exams should be given only after employment is offered, and then appropriate accommodations for individuals with disabilities should be made. This process is not only fair, it also assures organizations that they will not be deprived of competent workers because of stereotypes about the qualifications and capabilities of people with disabilities. The ADA covers appropriate questions for interviews and proper ways to keep confidential information that is revealed by those hired. Organizations intent on compliance with this complicated law should have regular training for anyone interviewing applicants.

Evaluation and Promotion

Evaluation and promotion are much the same as hiring from an ethical perspective. Fairness to employees and the interests of the organization actually converge on the idea of finding the most appropriate way to determine who is the best-qualified candidate. Unfortunately, other considerations are also involved. Employees generally believe that seniority should play a part in promotion decisions and that they ought to be rewarded for years of service to the organization. Organizations also have an interest in providing opportunities for promotion to their employees since this practice motivates achievement and encourages valued employees to remain with the firm. In their widely read analysis of long-term organizational success, *Built to Last*, James Collins and Jerry Porras point to "home-grown management" as one of the basic characteristics of the corporations they identify as successful or "visionary." They conclude:

> In short, it is not the quality of leadership that most separates the visionary companies [the subject of their study] from the comparison companies. It is the *continuity* of quality leadership that matters—continuity that preserves the core. Both the visionary companies and the comparison companies have had excellent top management at certain points in their histories. But the visionary companies have had better management development and succession planning. . . . They thereby ensured greater continuity of leadership talent grown from within than the comparison companies in fifteen out of eighteen cases.
>
> (Collins and Porras, 1997: 173–174)

Visionary companies, according to Collins and Porras, also have well-established evaluation and promotion processes that do not rely on seniority alone. Where the senior employee is also the most qualified, there may be no problem with selection from within the organization. But this is not always the case; sometimes employees have seniority at their current level because they have not been offered employment by other organizations.

Clear organizational policies regarding the role of seniority in evaluation and promotion decisions can help to clarify the problem, but the basic dilemma of seniority versus merit will remain. There are important values on both sides. For the organization itself, maintaining employee morale and building loyalty weigh in favor of seniority as an important criterion, while efficiency may at times weigh against it. Human resource managers should be aware that consistent hiring from outside the organization to fill upper-level vacancies can deflate morale among middle-level employees with abilities and ambition. Even on the level of organizational policy, there is no easy resolution to this matter. According to William H. Shaw of San Jose State University,

> Of paramount importance in any decision is that management remember its twin responsibilities of promoting on the basis of qualifications and of recognizing prolonged and constructive contributions to the firm. A policy that provides for promotions strictly on the basis of qualifications seems heartless, whereas one that promotes by seniority alone seems mindless.
>
> (Shaw, 1991:203)

While people may deserve opportunities based on their years of service, and while the organization may find it good management policy to emphasize employee development and promotion from within, seniority cannot be considered a fundamental right.

Dismissal

With respect to discipline or discharge, the moral right to fair treatment implies that employees will be disciplined or terminated only for just cause, that is, that they will not be judged on the basis of non-job-related criteria. Job-related considerations include insubordination, incompetence, infractions of organizational rules, absenteeism, misuse or misappropriation of organizational property, and dereliction of duty. Organizations that are too lenient in these matters risk establishing a culture that undermines staff morale. Ethically, respect for individuals implies that decisions affecting their livelihood will not be made arbitrarily. Due process is a guarantee of fair treatment. It is often a major feature of union contracts, but it is equally important for nonunion employees. At a minimum, due process involves an opportunity to respond to charges and to have important employment decisions reviewed at higher levels of management.

Firing employees is a complex ethical action. It is often thought that since the organization has no more interest in the employee, the quickest termination, or the least costly, or the least disruptive internally must be the best. Employees are told not to report the next day on their way out the door one evening, or called at home and told that they are terminated effective immediately, or rushed through a consultant's office and escorted back to their desk to pick up personal items before being shown to the door. This inconsiderate treatment is often explained as necessary to protect the organization. But it can actually make a difficult situation worse, not only for the employee being dismissed, but also for other employees and for managers who have to make the decisions and take the actions. Employees are always aware of and sensitive to the manner in which a colleague is dismissed, and imagine that they might well be treated the same way themselves—which, of course, may be true. If there is no warning and no opportunity to close relationships, or even to prepare oneself mentally and emotionally, the shock sent through the organization is all the more damaging. It is like reacting to a death. The expected death of a loved one is difficult enough; an unexpected death is always more traumatic and often leaves friends and relatives with a sense of unknown and imminent danger.

Warren Radtke, a Boston consultant on outplacement, points out that to understand the employee's situation, it is important to appreciate the sense of loss of control (Warren R. Radtke, 1999, personal communication). When someone is fired, the immediate consequence is that his or her ability to control this major life function (and probably other personal matters as well) virtually disappears. If dismissed employees can have some input into the process and some control over the actual course of events, therefore, the more they and their coworkers will be able to deal with the shock. Escorting a person to the door, according to Radtke, is usually not necessary. Stated organizational policies, including time for personal adjustment and assistance with the resulting financial problems, can minimize the effects of dismissal and give assurances of fairness and humane treatment to employees who are retained.

As a by-product of the restructuring and downsizing of corporations in the United States in the past decade, there is now an extensive body of literature on human resource management practices regarding reductions in force. Daniel Kingsley's analysis, for example, shows sensitivity to the effect of a termination on the person who has the task of firing someone. Even the "terminator" often suspects, as one of Kingsley's sources said, that "what he does to one of his people today will happen to him later on," so the terminator's situation is equally stressful (Kingsley, 1984:25). This is not the place to recount the practical advice given by Kingsley and others (The New York Times, Inc., 1996; Wright and Smye, 1996) or to criticize the legalistic and defensive posture taken by many current textbook writers. My purpose is to point out that the worker being fired is nonetheless a person with moral rights and justifiable expectations as a stakeholder in the organization. The way an organization treats its employees even as they are being dismissed is a measure of its moral integrity.

PRIVACY

The notion of employee rights includes respect for their personal privacy. The acceptance of employment involves an agreement to act in certain ways—to be present for work, to perform assigned tasks, and to uphold to the interests of the organization. People do not give up their other rights, however, when they become employees. They retain their fundamental human rights, and among these is the right to privacy, which, according to many philosophers, stems from the right to life and liberty. The right to privacy covers both nonwork behavior and reasonable personal privacy while on the job.

Expectations regarding employees' off-the-job behavior are more important for professional and public service organizations than for industrial or business firms with little or no public exposure. Professional associations often attempt to set standards of personal conduct for their members, but these can change dramatically according to time and place. In years past, it was considered improper for physicians and nurses (as well as members of the clergy and teachers) to be involved in political activities, for example, but this is no longer the case. Off-the-job behavior such as drug or alcohol abuse that affects work performance can be a legitimate organizational concern, however, although this has to be balanced against the extent of organizational intrusion into personal lives.

Social norms are changing. It is now widely considered inappropriate for organizations to intrude on people's private lives at work as well. Workplace telephone and personal conversations, computer files, and personal papers are now commonly thought to be private. Employee privacy may also be protected by state law. In addition to regulations assuring the confidentiality of medical information, California law, for example, contains an Invasion of Privacy Act that states:

> Every person who, intentionally and without the consent of all parties to a confidential communication, by means of any electronic amplifying or recording device, eavesdrops upon or records the confidential communication, whether the communication is carried on among the parties in the presence of one another or by means of a telegraph, telephone, or other device, except a radio, shall be punished by a fine not exceeding two thousand five hundred dollars ($2,500), or imprisonment in the county jail not exceeding one year. . . . The term "confidential communication" includes any communication carried on in circumstances as may reasonably indicate that any party to the communication desires it to be confined to the parties thereto. . . .
>
> (California, 1990)

Dress codes that express personal identity are sometimes at issue. The extent to which employees should conform to a corporate or professional image on the job is debatable, but it should not simply be assumed that conformity to some top administrator's idea of proper appearance must prevail. Participation in wellness programs may also be viewed by some employees as intrusive. Compulsory programs educating workers about stress, nutrition, smoking, exercise, and other health-related matters may be justified by the organization's general concern for its employees' health, but may actually be private matters to some employees.

With healthcare organizations the issue of community reputation is sometimes problematic. Should an employee be fired for getting into a fight and being arrested, for disturbing the peace, or for soliciting the services of a pros-titute? The public image of the organization may be involved, but administra-tors should avoid drawing conclusions on these matters too quickly. Many problems with employee privacy are just practical matters that require a mea-sure of common sense. Consider, for example, the many dimensions of the following case.

Case 10.1 Privacy Accommodations

Paul Olson is 33 years old; he has a bachelor's degree in biology and a master's in biochemistry. Answering an advertisement in the *Washington Post*, Paul applied for a position as a sales representative/technical consultant with Krohl International, a major manufacturer of medical equipment. Krohl makes both external devices (meters and valves for artificial ventilators) and implantation devices such as pacemakers.

The position required a high degree of technical competence, which Paul had gained from his six years as a technical assistant with a pharmaceutical company. In the consul-tant position with Krohl, he would be meeting and talking with customers (physicians and technicians) and would be making presentations at medical conferences. He was very personable, well liked, and highly respected for his expertise.

Rudy Schwartz, Krohl's Director of Operations for the Washington, D.C., office, took an immediate liking to Paul. It was very difficult to find people with his background. It would take little time for Paul to learn the business, and Paul's references indicated that he would be a good consultant. The Krohl office in Washington is small. There are five sales consultants including Schwartz, who manages the office, two secretaries, and a receptionist.

When Paul was offered the job and Rudy explained the necessary paperwork to bring him on board, Paul told Rudy in confidence that he had been under a psychiatrist's care for five years and that he took regular medication. He said he would report this on the medical background form but wanted to let Rudy know. Rudy thanked him and asked if he thought this would affect his work in any way. Paul said that the only difficulty he would have would occur if there were any high-stress situations.

Rudy told Paul that almost all of the work involved rather low-key technical assist-ance and that the sales part involved no pressure. Krohl stood on its reputation as a leader with much of its equipment, and its marketing approach emphasized technical competence—just what Paul could do best. There was, however, an occasional online assistance request when technical consultants would be asked to assist with the use of new equipment at surgical procedures to make sure that the devices were functioning properly when implanted. This involved the scrub and gear of operating rooms, and there were some very critical situations. Paul doubted that he would handle such situations well.

Rudy was convinced that Paul was the person he wanted for the job, however, and suggested that he could easily assign the online requests to other members of the staff or take them himself. Paul took the job. The first five months went fine. Paul's expertise made him a valued addition to the unit. Rudy even began to give him the major confer-ence presentation tasks, and the other representatives agreed that he could field questions better than anyone. Then one of the technical consultants, Andy Cramer, noticed that Paul had never been assigned any of the online requests. He mentioned it to the other consultants, who said they had also been aware of this. Some of them eventually began to ask Paul about this and even to tease him for avoiding what they called the "gory details" of the work. When the teasing persisted, Rudy, the only person in the office who understood Paul's situation, wondered if this could become a problem and what he could do about it.

There was also the matter of the phone bill. Kohl had installed a new phone system at its Washington, D.C., office. The new system recorded all incoming and outgoing calls by phone extension, keeping the time, date, and duration of each call, the number calling or called, and the party. Conversations were not recorded, only the accounting information. The new system provided a monthly printout by extension, dividing the calls into two categories: Customer (i.e., numbers on the office contact list) and Other.

When the first report came in, Gail Carrier, the receptionist, brought it to Rudy. Some sales consultants had confined their calls almost entirely to customers; others had longer lists of "Other" calls, many of which were to spouses or relatives. None of the "Other" calls, involved much time. But while discussing the report with Rudy, Gail, who was known for keeping track of people's business, noted that Paul Olson had placed about two calls a week to Psychiatric Services, Inc. "He must go there," she said. "I know his wife doesn't work there; she's at this other number."

This case raises a number of privacy issues. First, the matter of Paul's disability was handled well. He had disclosed his condition after the position was offered to him, and Rudy had suggested an appropriate accommodation. There was apparently no need to disclose this to the other employees. Paul's apparent exemption from online assistance and the inadvertent disclosure of his calls to the psychiatrist led to the problem. While there are many effective approaches to each of these problems (and a number of ineffective approaches as well), from the perspective of employee confidence it would seem appropriate for Paul to be consulted before any action is taken. His privacy is at stake, and he should be involved in finding a solution. He could, in fact, propose a solution that might not have occurred to his boss, such as disclosing his disability to his colleagues.

Drug Testing

Drug testing has been a controversial issue in the workplace in recent years, although it has now become an accepted practice in some industries where life and safety are at risk. Drug testing programs vary widely in nature and scope. Testing all employees on an annual basis has proved ineffective and generally has little or no relationship to work requirements. It is also illegal in a number of states except for employees in certain job categories. Random testing of employees who are in positions of responsibility for actions that might endanger themselves or others is more effective and is now accepted as a necessary evil, although determining which employees are in such positions is still a matter of debate. If a risk of direct harm to individuals (coworkers, clients, or others) is involved, testing may become relatively routine. If only loss of productivity with no risk of personal harm is the concern, there is less justification for testing. When an employee's productivity or absenteeism is the problem, it may best be treated as a matter of work performance. Testing subsequent to work incidents or on suspicion of supervisors (with evidence of impaired performance) can be effective, but this requires what amounts to an accusation of misconduct. In any case, drug testing always involves a number of concerns related to respect for employees as individuals, including sensitivity to personal privacy, the security and confidentiality of test results, checks for false-positive tests, and employee assistance and medical programs. Literature on the details of drug testing programs is now extensive and widely available (BNA, 1998).

As with most employment practices, the perception of fairness is crucial. Drug testing always intrudes on the privacy of employees and can contribute to a climate of distrust. This negative effect can be overcome, however, if the rationale for a drug testing program is clearly laid out. To state the obvious, drug testing is not necessary if there is no reason for it, so the first question to ask is whether there is evidence that warrants the intrusion. If it becomes clear that a testing program is necessary and this is made clear to employees, the program will stand a good chance of being accepted. The best evidence of the necessity for a testing program would be the number of tests based on suspicion that were required in the organization's recent history. Testing everyone is a poor way to address problems with one individual. Employee involvement in the development of a program is essential.

WHISTLE-BLOWING

Employees who expose organizational wrongdoing can generally expect to be mistreated themselves (Boatright, 1997; De George, 1990). The overwhelming evidence from studies of whistle-blowing is that those who take the step of reporting illegal or unethical activities are likely to be ostracized, criticized, shut out, abused, passed over for promotions, or fired (Miceli and Near, 1992; Westin, 1981). And whistle-blowers usually have little or no recourse. In fact, those who choose to disclose wrongdoing would be well advised to be prepared to seek employment with a new company, if not in a new field. Corporations simply don't like people who expose their mistakes. The irony of this situation is that organizations really need to know what is happening within their walls so that problems can be corrected (Baab and Ozar, 1994; Callahan and Dworkin, 1991). They need to avoid legal liability and to stop misuse of organizational resources, so they have an interest in discovering what is going on, even though they often punish employees for disclosing it.

Two types of whistle-blowing can be distinguished: internal and external. Internal whistle-blowing is reporting wrongdoing, whether it is an illegal act or actions contrary to the interests of the organization, to authorities within the organization itself. The disclosure can be made to direct supervisors, to superiors above those to whom one reports directly, to legal counsel, to an internal auditor, or to a compliance officer. External whistle-blowing is reporting wrong-doing to public authorities or to the media. Since employees owe loyalty to the organizations in which they work, it is generally thought that they have an obligation to report wrongdoing internally before going to legal authorities or to the public. In any case, the decision to expose wrongdoing on the part of fellow employees or superiors, or wrongdoing of the organization itself (practices known to and condoned by individuals at the highest levels), is a difficult one. A few simple principles may be helpful in deciding when whistle-blowing is justified:

- internal means of solving the problem should be exhausted prior to going to legal authorities or to the media,
- the person blowing the whistle should have sufficient evidence of the wrongdoing,
- the harm or potential harm must be serious enough to outweigh harm to the organization from the exposure of its actions,
- the harm or potential harm must be imminent, and
- exposure of the wrongdoing must not be motivated by vengeance against individuals or the organization itself.

Some commentators also say that the benefit to others or to the organization itself should outweigh the consequences that the whistle-blower and his or her family are likely to suffer. This is indeed a consideration; the risk cannot be overemphasized. There are times when whistle-blowing would be morally justi-fied, but the individual should not feel morally obligated to take the risk. Rich-ard De George (1990) offers an extended analysis of the distinction between "morally permitted" and "morally required" whistle-blowing.

Case 10.2 Whistle-Blowing

Grace Miller, a registered nurse, is a billing auditor for a 180-bed rural hospital. Her job is to review medical records and to confirm charges for services performed. While much of this activity is routine, when discrepancies appear it is her duty to identify them and call them to the attention of her superior. The supervisor then checks with the physician, unit clerk, or nurse to determine exactly what services were ordered and whether they were provided. In some cases, this is also a question of what equipment was used.

When Miller was new to the job, she thought that her supervisor had extensive knowl-edge of medical practice and the general procedures at the hospital. More recently, how-ever, she has begun to wonder about this. There seem to be times when her supervisor says she knows that some procedures are normal and that certain equipment is always used even though the medical records themselves are quite ambiguous. The supervisor seldom seems to check with physicians or nurses to confirm the charges. More than once, when Miller asked about a charge for a procedure or the supplies used, she was simply told to bill the more expensive supplies because "that's what they always use," even though she knew from other records that less expensive procedures and supplies were used quite often. Eventually, she realized that her supervisor was simply resolving all ambiguities in favor of the most expensive alternatives. This may have increased hospital revenues, but it was certainly contrary to standard accounting practice and, she thought, contrary to the accuracy the hospital owed to its patients and its payers. The more Miller questioned her supervisor about this, however, the more annoyed the supervisor became. Finally, she told Miller that this was the way it had always been done, that the Billing Department couldn't bother the doctors and nurses about these details, and that there were certainly enough services and supplies used that were not recorded to make up the difference. The announcement of a new compliance program at the hospital, however, made Miller think that this was perhaps the type of situation that should be reported.

It can probably be assumed that no one is in any physical danger because of this situation, so Miller has time to consider her actions. How much evidence should she have before doing anything? Stories of things that happen normally without specific instances may not be very convincing to her superiors. But collecting specific evidence to report would have the effect of making Miller an investigator. Even with sufficient evidence, she would have to decide how to report the problem. Should she report the problem to the new compliance officer or go to her supervisor's superior informally? It would hardly seem justified for her to report the practice to federal inspectors without first bringing it to the attention of hospital officials. Finally, how can she avoid getting labeled untrustworthy if she reports this? She may not be able to avoid this at all, regardless of the outcome of the matter.

A few states have enacted laws to protect whistle-blowers from retaliation, but most laws cover only the public sector. In a 1968 case the U.S. Supreme Court affirmed the right of a public employee to criticize the government agency that employed him as long as a public interest in the matter was at stake (Pickering, 1968). In 1978 this right was extended to private contractors who work for the government (Holodnak, 1975), but the right is still based on the fact that there is a public interest involved. One argument against legal whistle-blowing protection is that employees may find excuses to blow the whistle when they feel that they are about to be fired or laid off and then claim protection against being discharged (Westin, 1981). It has also been argued that litigation over whistle-blowing would create an adversarial climate that would inhibit cooperation in the workplace. And it has been suggested that a legal remedy involving reinstatement would put an employee who is perceived as disloyal back in the workplace (Boatright, 1997). These arguments have all been raised against civil rights laws at various times, however, and for the most part have been found to be without merit.

Increasingly, organizations are developing policies on whistle-blowing that attempt to give the organization itself the benefit of having wrongdoing reported while at the same time protecting employees who make such reports. Effective reporting procedures can be difficult to establish, however. Employees have to believe that the procedures for investigation will be effective and will not leave them exposed to retaliation. Policies and procedures for investigations need to be explicit; employees have a right to know how any report of wrong-doing will be treated. Guarantees against retaliation can never be absolute, and this should be made clear to employees at the outset. Internally, investigations must include interviews with employees, and ultimately, decisions must be based on facts. When litigation is involved, furthermore, those accused of wrongdoing have a right to face their accusers. The accuser should be the organization itself, but the organization cannot establish its case without testimony from specific employees. Legal discovery and depositions can always override promises of confidentiality. What is important to most employees, however, is that the organization will stand by the employees who report illegal activities or wrongdoing.

If the corporate culture has no effective grievance or feedback procedures, employees are likely to appeal to the public interest. This can lead to calls for legislation: the 105th Congress saw the introduction of a Patient Safety and Health Care Whistleblower Protection Act to prohibit discrimination or retaliation against healthcare workers who report unsafe conditions and practices that affect patient care. The bill provides that

> (a) No person shall retaliate or discriminate in any manner against any health care worker because the worker (or any person acting on behalf of the worker) in good faith—
> (1) engaged in any disclosure of information relating to the care, services, or conditions of a health care entity;
> (2) advocated on behalf of a patient or patients with respect to the care, services, or conditions of a health care entity; or
> (3) initiated, cooperated, or otherwise participated in any investigation or proceeding of any governmental entity relating to the care, services, or conditions of a health care entity.
>
> (HR3342, 1998)

Employees in healthcare organizations have a special interest in whistle-blowing mechanisms and protection against retaliation. They see themselves as care providers and want to maintain the integrity of their work. Many now feel that they need to protect themselves and their patients from corporate cost-cutting that places patients at risk and overburdens staff. An effective whistle-blowing mechanism can be an important safety valve in difficult times.

UNIONS AND UNION AVOIDANCE

The right by which employers are free to associate (and to form corporations) for their mutual benefit is the same right by which workers are free to organize and bargain collectively to advance their interests. In a society based on the liberty of individuals, the government has a duty not to interfere with union organizing unless the welfare of society is at stake. This can happen, but again, the same rule applies to employers and employees. Agreements between corporations to fix prices or control markets can be contrary to the public good. Strikes or agreements among workers to withhold labor can also be contrary to the public good if this harms people directly or constitutes a conspiracy to drive up the price of labor. Social welfare notwithstanding, the right of workers to organize is specifically mentioned in the Universal Declaration of Human Rights (UN, 1948). The right to strike, as long as employees have not entered into an agreement to the contrary, is simply an extension of this right.

The pros and cons of trade union representation in the healthcare industry are widely debated. Many healthcare administrators are adamantly opposed to unions, believing that they undermine the cooperative nature of a workplace which is dependent on close employee relations. Many employees also see their work as professional in a sense that makes trade union organization unnecessary and even counterproductive. Others feel that they are so much at the mercy of the organizations for which they work that they must organize if they are to have any power as stakeholders at all.

Many healthcare organizations have established union avoidance programs to counter employees' efforts to organize. These programs often use employee surveys to gauge worker satisfaction, establish employee councils to discuss issues, and set pay scales equal to or above regional industry standards. Healthcare organizations often see these programs as pro-employee rather than anti-union (Professional Labor Relations Services, Inc., 1998). While this motivation might be questioned, such programs can sometimes be quite responsive to employees' interests.

The opposite side of the coin is that employees may never be sufficiently empowered without an independent organization. Regardless of how employee-centered an organization may be, any employee empowerment program that is ultimately under the control of organizational administrators smacks of the fox guarding the chicken coop. Whether organizations themselves can create mechanisms to empower workers is debatable, but the opportunity for employees to have an independent organization does enforce their power as stakeholders, giving them greater organizational representation. On the other hand, if unions take an exclusively adversarial stance, the culture of the organization can become locked in partisan dispute that substitutes grievance boards and arbitration for cooperative mechanisms.

OCCUPATIONAL HEALTH AND SAFETY

One issue with a long history in employee relations is occupational health and safety. Safety is an undeniable human right—an integral element of life and liberty in any meaningful sense of these terms. Many jobs, however, entail unavoidable risk. If risk cannot be eliminated entirely, however, it must be minimized.

Healthcare organizations are not the safest places to work. According to the Service Employees International Union, nursing home work is now one the most dangerous occupations (SEIU, 1997):

> Between 1984 and 1995, the illness and injury rate increased from 11.6 to 18.2 per 100 full-time workers, a 57 percent increase, with more than 200,000 injuries reported in the industry every year. This rate is considerably higher than the 1995 incidence of injury in industries traditionally considered high risk such as coal mining (6.2), construction (10.6), blast furnaces and steel mills (11.9), warehousing and trucking (13.8) and paper mills (7.5).
>
> (McDonald and Muller, 1998:4)

Workers' rights to health and safety must be protected by law. In a free market system, those employers who do nothing to protect the health and safety of their workers will theoretically be able to sell their goods and services at lower prices, so one employer cannot take effective steps to minimize health and safety risks to employees unless other employers do the same. The right to reasonable health and safety measures, therefore, requires government regulation. The federal Occupational Safety and Health Act (OSHA) of 1970 thus requires employers to keep the workplace "free from recognized hazards that are causing or are likely to cause death or serious injury" (OSHA, 1970). This federal standard, however, is neither clear nor absolute. What is to count as a hazard is debatable; whether certain substances pose a threat to health is unknown in some cases; and whether routine actions required in many jobs constitute ergonomic hazards is difficult to determine. The law also stipulates that the workplace is to be maintained free from hazards "to the maximum extent practicable." It is clear that some dangers simply cannot be eliminated, but this also leaves room for the question of whether reduction of risk beyond a certain point is financially feasible.

Under OSHA, the Department of Labor sets regulations and requirements for workplace health and safety. Most healthcare organizations have extensive compliance and training programs to conform to OSHA requirements. Some of these may seem overly cautious, redundant, or unnecessary; but there are other hazards that are still unregulated. Apart from OSHA workplace requirements, healthcare organizations face the question of infectious disease control. Guidelines in this area are set by the federal Centers for Disease Control and by the JCAHO.

Despite these extensive rules and regulations, healthcare workers are still injured on the job or become ill from exposure to toxic substances or infections, thus raising the question of liability. Theoretically, employers are not liable for injuries when workers are negligent. If a worker's own negligence is a contributory cause of an accident, the organization's liability is reduced to that extent. A second defense against organizational liability for injuries or health problems is that it may be impossible or impractical to make the workplace any safer than it is. The presence of minimal levels of carcinogenic substances is a good example. The absolute elimination of certain chemicals known to be carcinogenic from the workplace would, in some cases, *raise* the likelihood of exposure to other hazards. It has been notably difficult for federal agencies such as the Environmental Protection Agency to set minimal safe exposure levels to many substances. Hazards that cannot be eliminated fall under the common-law concept of the *voluntary assumption of risk.* Healthcare workers know that if a patient falls, for example, a caregiver may injure herself in attempting to save the patient from injury. Jobs in health care entail certain unavoidable risks, and people know this when they seek employment.

Corporate defense lawyers often seek to deny organizational liability by claiming either worker negligence or the voluntary assumption of risk. This is part of our adversarial legal system, and lawyers are charged with defending the interests of organizations, which they have traditionally viewed as financial interests. From an ethical perspective, however, organizations have a much wider range of interests. They must consider the interests of their employees. Separating the interests of the organization per se from those of its employees is both artificial and unwise. The acceptance of responsibility for workplace injuries and hazards is a matter of trust between employers and workers, not just a matter of legal liability. Trust involves reasonable expectations between employers and employees and requires a willingness to cooperate in order to find solutions to problems. So, above and beyond strict legal liabilities, healthcare administrators need to decide what their moral obligations to workers imply. This may include accepting "no-fault" responsibility or offering assistance in situations where the organization is not legally liable. Many human resource managers can point to instances in which healthcare organizations have voluntarily accepted responsibility for workplace injuries and have assisted employees and their families even when they could have claimed that the worker was negligent.

Trust between employees and the organizations for which they work implies honesty, which in turn means disclosing all information that employees need to decide whether or not to risk their safety or health given the unavoidable hazards of the workplace. Workers can thus be said to have a right to know what risks they are taking. Employers have a corresponding duty to tell workers about these risks, if they know, and a duty to take reasonable steps to find out what they don't know. This does raise questions, however. Do employees have a right to know about exposure to toxic substances that took place in the past if that risk was only recently discovered? Do ex-employees have a right to know? And at what level of risk, or possible risk, should employees be informed?

Despite the difficulties, employees' right to know about workplace hazards is a strong ethical requirement. Lack of knowledge effectively deprives people of their freedom. Without knowing the risks involved, workers cannot judge whether to accept a job, request protective equipment, apply for a transfer, or look for a new position. This is a matter of informed consent comparable to the informed consent of patients in clinical settings. The standard for disclosure, furthermore, should be high. Faden and Beauchamp argue that the standard should not be professional or technical.

> These problems center on communication rather than on legal standards of disclosure. The key to effective communication is to invite participation by workers in a dialogue. . . . Different levels of education, linguistic ability, and sophistication about the issues need to be accommodated.
>
> (Faden and Beauchamp, 1997:219)

The OSHA regulations on disclosure of workplace hazards are now extensive (OSHA, 1998). They include employee notification through container labeling and material safety data sheets, required training programs, required protective devices, and the right of workers to request OSHA inspections. The practice of making material safety data sheets available for employee inspection is a good example of an ethical obligation. The data sheets themselves may be technically correct, but if they are not clear and helpful, employees may not bother to consult them. So healthcare organizations that are concerned about employee use of hazardous materials may need to find other ways to inform their employees about potential dangers. The ethical obligation extends beyond regulatory requirements.

Employee safety is an important element of organizational integrity. No aspect of organizational activities demonstrates the organization's attitude toward its employees more directly or more constantly than its concern for their health and safety. If an organization wants to build employee trust and cooperation, there is no better place to start than with an interactive and effective program for health and safety. "Safety Alert" or "Safety Concern" reports, separate from OSHA complaints and the organizational compliance hotline, have been successful in many organizations because they draw the attention of safety managers to problems without the risks of higher-level whistle-blowing.

Other aspects of employee health and safety can be problematic, especially chronic physical conditions resulting from long-term, repetitive job activities. The constant use of video display terminals, for instance, is known to cause eye strain, blurred vision, repetitive motion problems, back pain, and shoulder and neck distress. Dental hygienists and other direct caregivers face similar problems of neck and back strain due to repetitive positioning and motion. In general, employers do a better job with safety measures (although the incidence of accidents is still high) and with notification about hazardous materials (although there is still much that is not known here) than with long-range health problems due to exposure or poor ergonomics. Some of these problems raise the question of employers' right to track workers' medical conditions. Again, a cooperative and communicative employer–employee approach is the best way to demonstrate organizational concern.

CONCLUSIONS

There is a wide spectrum of attitudes among administrators and governing boards toward employee relations. At one extreme is the view that employees have to be dealt with effectively in order to fulfill the organization's basic goals. In the middle of the spectrum is the notion that employees are crucial to the operation of any service organization—"our most important asset," as some mission statements put it. And at the other end of the spectrum is the view that employees' well-being itself is one of the many goals of the organization, that providing fulfilling and creative work along with opportunities for advancement and appropriate compensation is an integral part of the mission of the organization. The last, I would say, is the moral ideal; it accepts employees as primary stakeholders along with patients, administrators, and the community. This focus is not always easy to maintain, however. Even the phrase *employee relations*— the title of this chapter—could be taken to imply that there is an organization on the one hand that relates to a group of employees on the other. Human resource managers can play an important role in achieving and maintaining an ideal focus, provided that they see their professional mandate as representing the employees to the administrators, as well as speaking to the employees on behalf of the administration.

REFERENCES

AHA (American Hospital Association), 1998, *Hospital Statistics 1998*, Chicago: American Hospital Association.

Baab, David A., and David T. Ozar, 1994, "Whistleblowing in Dentistry: What Are the Ethical Issues?" *Journal of the American Dental Association*, 125:199–205.

BNA (Bureau of National Affairs, Inc.), 1983, "Employee Selection Procedures," *ASPA-BNA Survey No. 45*, http://www.bna.com/ (12/13/98).

———, 1998, "Human Resources Library on the Web," http://www.bna.com/mkt/hrl/hrl-wdesc.htm (1/6/99).

Boatright, John R., 1997, *Ethics and the Conduct of Business*, Upper Saddle River, NJ: Prentice-Hall.

California, 1990, California Penal Code, Invasion of Privacy Act, §632, Eavesdropping On or Recording Confidential Communications (Amended by Stats. 1990, c. 696 (A.B. 3457) §3.

Callahan, Elleta Sangrey, and Terry Morehead Dworkin, 1991, "Internal Whistleblowing: Protecting the Interests of the Employee, the Organization, and Society," *American Business Law Journal*, 29(2):267–308.

Caudron, Shari, 1996, "Rebuilding Employee Trust," *Training and Development*, 50(8): 18–21.

Chruden, Herbert J., and Arthur W. Sherman, Jr., 1984, *Managing Human Resources*, 7th ed., Cincinnati: South-Western Publishing Company.

Collins, James L., and Jerry Porras, 1997, *Built to Last*, New York: HarperCollins Publishers.

Columbus (Columbus Community Hospital), 1998, "Columbus Community Hospital," http://www.columbuscommunity.com/ (1/3/99).

De George, Richard, T., 1990, *Business Ethics*, 3rd ed., New York: Macmillan Publishing Company.

Dessler, Gary, 1997, *Human Resource Management*, Upper Saddle River, NJ: Prentice-Hall.

Epstein, Richard A., 1984, "In Defense of the Contract at Will," *University of Chicago Law Review*, 51(4):947–982.

Faden, Ruth R., and Tom L. Beauchamp, 1997, "The Right to Risk Information and the Right to Refuse Workplace Hazards, in Tom L. Beauchamp, and Norman E. Bowie, eds., *Ethical Theory and Business*, 5th ed., Upper Saddle River, NJ: Prentice-Hall.

Griggs, 1971, *Griggs v. Duke Power Company*, 401 U.S. 424.

Holodnak, 1975, *Holodnak v. Avco Corporation*, 514 *F*. 2nd 285.

HR3342, 1998, "Patient Safety and Health Care Whistleblower Protection Act of 1998," http://thomas.loc.gov/ (12/5/99).

Hunter, John H., and Rhonda Hunter, 1984, "The Validity and Utility of Alternative Predictors of Job Performance," *Psychological Bulletin*, 96:72–98.

Kingsley, Daniel T., 1984, *How to Fire an Employee*, New York: Facts on File Publications.

Lochner, 1905, *Lochner v. New York*, 198 U.S. 45; 25 S.Ct. 539.

McDonald, Ingrid, and Arvid Muller, 1998, *The Staffing Crisis in Nursing Homes: Why It's Getting Worse and What Can Be Done About It*, Washington, DC: Service Employees International Union.

Miceli, Marcia P., and Janet P. Near, 1992, *Blowing the Whistle: The Organizational and Legal Implications for Companies and Employees*, New York: Lexington Books.

Milkovich, George T., and John W. Boudreau, 1988, *Personnel/Human Resource Management*, 5th ed., Homewood, IL: Richard D. Irwin.

OSHA (Occupational Safety and Health Act), 1970, Occupational Safety and Health Act, Sec. 5(a)(1).

OSHA (Occupational Safety and Health Administration), 1998, "Employee Workplace Rights and Responsibilities," Fact Sheet No. OSHA 91–35, http://www.lectlaw.com/files/emp30 (12/30/98).

Paine, 1884, *Paine v. Western & A.R.R.*, 81 Tenn. 507.

Pickering, 1968, *Pickering v. Board of Education*, 391 U.S. 563.

Professional Labor Relations Services, Inc., 1998, "Professional Labor Relations Services," http://www.unionavoidance.com (12/18/98).

Scanlon, T. M., 1977, "Due Process," in J. Roland Pennock and John W. Chapman, eds., *Nomos XVIII: Due Process*, New York: New York University Press.

SEIU (Service Employees International Union), 1997, "Caring Til It Hurts: How Nursing

Home Work Is Becoming the Most Dangerous Job in America," Washington, DC: Service Employee International Union.

Shaw, William H. 1991, *Business Ethics*, Belmont, CA: Wadsworth Publishing Company.

The New York Times, Inc., 1996, *The Downsizing of America*, New York: Random House.

UN (United Nations), 1948, "Universal Declaration of Human Rights" (G.A. res. 217A (III), U.N. Doc A/810 at 71), http://www.udhr50.org/UDHR/default.htm (12/16/99).

Velasquez, Manuel G., 1998, *Business Ethics: Concepts and Cases*, 4th ed., Upper Saddle River, NJ: Prentice-Hall.

Werhane, Patricia H., 1985, *Persons, Rights and Corporations*, Englewood Cliffs, NJ: Prentice-Hall.

Westin, Alan F., 1981, *Whistle Blowing! Loyalty and Dissent in the Corporation*, New York: McGraw-Hill.

Wright, Lesley, and Marti Smye, 1996, *Corporate Abuse*, New York: Macmillan Publishing Company.

11

CLINICAL ETHICS, MEDICAL RESEARCH, AND COMPLIANCE PROGRAMS

This chapter deals with three common programs of healthcare organizations that are closely related to organizational ethics: clinical ethics committees, institutional review boards for medical research, and compliance programs. Each has a mandate that is focused on ethical considerations; but each has its own jurisdiction. Only a brief introduction to the scope of these programs can be offered here, along with consideration of the ways in which each is related to organizational ethics.

CLINICAL MEDICAL ETHICS

Interest in clinical medical ethics emerged only in the 1950s and 1960s in the work of philosopher-theologians such as Joseph Fletcher (1955) and Paul Ramsey (1970). Public concern about human experimentation was aroused by Henry Beecher's (1966) exposé of research abuse in 1966 and by the 1972 revelation of the Tuskegee syphilis study (Pence, 1995). The first heart transplant and the selection of patients for kidney dialysis in the 1960s raised further questions. In the 1970s, the Quinlan case brought the issue of refusing life support to public attention, and the Tarasoff case in California raised the question of the confidentiality of medical information in the face of danger to others. It was the issues of informed consent to medical or surgical treatment and of withholding or withdrawing life-sustaining treatment, however, that brought ethical problems to the attention of almost every healthcare organization in the country. Hospitals felt compelled to develop policies on these issues to guide physicians and patients. Committees were then established to formulate policy and then to assist with difficult decisions.

Clinical ethics committees differ to a remarkable extent in their nature and scope. In many cases, these differences are a consequence of their origins: some were started by physicians as a forum for discussing difficult cases, others were started as patient service programs, and still others grew out of the organizational necessity to develop policies. These origins are often reflected in the activities of committees today. Some are closely related to medical staff, while others are more advisory to patients and their families. Originally, some ethics committees were assigned semi-legal functions, acting as juries to decide such difficult cases as withdrawing treatment or allocating organs for transplantation. This juridical function, however, has given way almost entirely to the notion of consultation. Hospital ethics committees now generally see themselves as advisory in nature—although advising can sometimes include conflict resolution.

Generally, hospital ethics committees are thought to have three functions:

1. Education of hospital staff members, patients, and the public about medical ethics, especially in regard to informed consent and advance directives.
2. Policy development for institutions regarding issues such as "do not resuscitate" orders and withholding or withdrawing life-sustaining treatment.
3. Consultation with physicians and patients to offer advice on a case-by-case basis.

The educational functions of hospital ethics committees may include regular meetings at which issues and cases are discussed, continuing education programs and conferences, involvement in medical school classroom or resident education, and the publication of materials for patients and their families. In the area of policy development, many clinical ethics committees are now finding that they need to revise institutional policies that were written in the 1980s or early 1990s. New policies are also being considered, especially in the areas of end-of-life care and medical futility (the conditions under which physicians and hospitals may refuse requests for treatment that offers little or no hope of medical benefit).

The Legal Context

Clinical ethics committees also typically have a strong interest in state laws that establish mandatory guidelines for clinical practice. Laws governing medical practice fall into certain generic types, which can be briefly outlined as follows:

1. *Informed consent.* In most states, this concept is found in court decisions rather than in statutes because it is an aspect of contract law. The purchasing and receiving of medical services represents a contract between a provider and a consumer. Since consumers (i.e., patients) are generally in no position to judge either their own medical needs or the potential benefits of any given treatment, courts have said that providers (i.e., physicians) must explain patients' medical conditions and must obtain fully informed consent from patients or their appointed surrogates before treating. Theoretically, this means that a physician must explain a patient's medical condition, proposed treatment, possible benefits and risks of treatment, available alternative treatments along with their risks and benefits, and, finally, what is likely to happen if the condition is left untreated. The legal standard for this explanation is the patient's need for information, not a professional judgment of whether the explanation was medically accurate.

2. *Living will.* Living will statutes vary from state to state. A living will, according to *Taber's Cyclopedic Medical Dictionary*, 17th edition, is a statement prepared at a time when an individual is capable of making his or her own decisions that "attests to the wish that heroic measures such as use of life support devices not be used to prolong life when it is obvious that such actions will not permit recovery from the condition" (Thomas, 1993:1129).

It can be difficult to determine whether a patient is capable of making his or her own end-of-life decision. Current opinion indicates that as long as there is no evidence of psychological conditions that would impair the patient's judgment, this should be a functional determination based on whether the patient understands the medical condition and is able to formulate and express his or her wishes rather than a psychological determination of the patient's mental status (Lo, 1995).

A living will is a specific form of advance directive. Advance directives generally state a competent person's preferences for treatment in the event that the person loses his or her capacity to decide later. The federal Patient Self-Determination Act passed in 1991 gives legal status to advance directives that go well beyond the terminal conditions indicated in many state living will statutes. Evidence to the contrary notwithstanding, it is now well established that patients' clearly and competently stated wishes for their health care should be followed.

3. *Medical power of attorney or medical agent laws.* These laws give people the right to appoint someone to make their medical decisions should they become unable to do so. In many states, the appointment of a surrogate decision maker requires a legal form with signatures and witnesses. This process can become needlessly cumbersome. Most people can specify readily who they would like to make such decisions, and this could be recorded by a physician doing an initial medical exam or by a nurse taking a patient's medical history.

The fact that some people need to give serious thought to the designation of a surrogate should be treated as a special case. The powers of a surrogate normally extend to all healthcare decisions, including the choice of a physician.

4. *Surrogate appointment.* A more recent type of law establishes rules under which a physician can appoint a surrogate decision maker for a patient who has not designated one. Typically these laws contain a priority list of surrogates (spouse, adult child, parent, sibling, etc.), but they also designate conditions under which the physician can appoint someone outside of the designated order if that person is better able to convey the patient's wishes. These laws make it unnecessary for physicians and hospitals to go to court to have a surrogate decision maker or guardian appointed. Both power-of-attorney and surrogate appointment laws generally indicate that the surrogate should make medical decisions first according to the patient's known wishes and second on the basis of the surrogate's opinion of the patient's best interests.

5. *"Do not resuscitate" laws.* Many states also have statutes giving physicians the right to order that cardiopulmonary resuscitation (CPR) not be attempted. This is generally the only case in which a physician needs to write an order *not* to do something; the reason, of course, is that in emergency situations it must be presumed that CPR will be given. So if CPR is not likely to be effective and the patient does not want it, an order to this effect—usually accompanied by an identification card or bracelet—is needed. "Do not resuscitate" laws in most states, however, require that the patient or the patient's family be notified and consent to the order. This is a reasonable protection of patient rights, but it also allows patients to insist on CPR in situations where there is no hope of medical benefit and the procedure is entirely futile.

Recently, laws have been passed in some states to protect physicians when they prescribe higher than average doses of pain medication. Further legislation regarding end-of-life care and physician-assisted suicide is under consideration in some states. Behind this legislation lies the general question of the extent to which medical practice ought to be specified in law. While earlier laws gave patients specific rights, recent laws have been passed to assist or protect physicians.

Ethics Consultation

Faced with the task of giving ethical guidance on medical decisions, bioethicists and members of clinical ethics committees in the 1980s attempted to develop of a set of general principles that could be applied to problem cases. Eventually, a loose but rather effective consensus emerged on a framework of basic principles reflected in influential textbooks (Beauchamp and Childress, 1994) and ethics committee guidelines (Hastings, 1987). The principles were typically described as *(1)* autonomy in terms of patient decision making, *(2)* beneficence or patients' well-being, *(3)* the integrity of healthcare professionals, and *(4)* justice in the distribution of healthcare resources. It was recognized that these principles often conflict with one another and that they do not provide a systematic process for the resolution of ethical dilemmas, but they provide some guidance nonetheless.

In the 1990s other ethical perspectives began to emerge, providing different insights. Feminist philosophers argued that the focus on principles gave ethical considerations a legalistic cast that did not well reflect the network of relationships and obligations that are essential to morality. Virtue theorists advanced considerations of motivation and character that went beyond the basic principles and narrative theorists drew attention to the ways in which medical decisions should reflect the development of a person's life and remain consistent with his or her "story." The effect of these trends has been to make medical ethics more case-centered and less rule-governed.

Many hospital ethics committees now offer case consultation as a regular service to patients and their families, as well as to physicians and nurses. The American Society for Bioethics and Humanities, a national professional association of medical ethicists, has developed a set of standards for such consultations (ASBH, 1998). Graduate programs, institutional centers, professional conferences, and a wealth of literature have made the field an active one. Medical ethics consultation is still not universally available, however, and ambiguities concerning its role still exist. In some places, consultation is clearly a service to patients and their families. In other places, it seems to serve the interests of physicians in gaining patients' compliance with professional treatment plans; that is, it may become a tool of the medical establishment (DeVries and Subedi, 1998).

Medical ethics is a complex field. Ethics committees now face new problems of offering services for outpatients and home health patients and of maintaining contact with patients who move through the various levels of a continuum of care (Christensen and Tucker, 1997). While consensus has developed on some issues, others are subject to considerable debate (Arras and Steinbock, 1999; Beauchamp and Walters, 1999; Thomasma and Kushner, 1996; Veatch, 1997; Wolf, 1996).

Healthcare administrators have two duties with respect to clinical ethics committees. The first is to see that they fulfill JCAHO standards for patients' rights and consultation services (JCAHO, 1996). A hospital ethics committee that is simply a subcommittee of the medical staff for the discussion of professional ethics issues might not satisfy the JCAHO standards very well in this respect. Second, healthcare organizations also have an interest in providing adequate clinical ethics policies for the guidance of physicians, nurses, and other caregivers. Those policies need to conform to state laws and to be consistent with the organization's mission statement. Policy development should be an orderly and effective administrative process in which all who have a stake are consulted.

Finally, the organizational ethics perspective raises the difficult question of justice in the distribution of healthcare resources. Clinical ethics committees have almost always been aware of justice issues, but they have seldom addressed them directly. It has even been a professional ideal in American society that healthcare decisions would be made in individual cases without regard to cost. The question of providing care that is considered medically futile, however, raises the issue of distributive justice in ways that clinical ethics committees and organizational administrators can hardly avoid (see Case 8.2 in Chapter 8). Even if the provision of futile care involves no moral wrong to the patient, the question of whether the patient has a right to whatever community resources his or her surrogate requests must be addressed directly.

Case 11.1 No Captain of the Ship

A number of clinical ethics problems require organizational solutions. One recurrent issue in some hospitals is the question of which member of a medical team is ultimately in charge of the ethical aspects of a case. The following case was written by Warren Point, M.D., one of the founding members of the clinical ethics committee at Massachusetts General Hospital.

Mr. S was a 42-year-old man, married, with two children 10 and 12 years old. He operated a small consulting firm and had minimal health insurance. He and his family had been very healthy, with no knowledge of any medical problems.

Mr. S developed a severe global headache suddenly one evening and lapsed immediately into a coma. On arrival at a nearby emergency room, he required tracheal intubation of his lungs and artificial ventilation. Examination revealed him to be totally unresponsive to stimuli. His blood pressure was markedly elevated. The findings of the neurological examination were consistent with massive brain damage. The lungs were slightly congested. Radiological examination of the brain revealed a massive hemorrhage displacing a significant amount of brain tissue. Chest x-rays were consistent with moderate lung congestion due to heart failure. The heart was enlarged in a manner suggesting prolonged high blood pressure. Laboratory data showed moderate kidney impairment. All other test results were within normal limits. There was no bleeding tendency.

The patient was admitted under the care of a neurosurgeon, who concluded that nothing could be done surgically to reverse the situation. Other physicians were consulted, including a heart specialist, a kidney specialist, a neurologist, a lung specialist, and Mr. S's own general physician, who had not seen the patient for several years.

After three weeks of no improvement, kidney dialysis was recommended. Mrs. S believed that her husband would not want to live in this state, which everyone agreed was irreversible. She asked the family doctor to stop treatment and allow her husband to die in peace. The family doctor replied that he could not allow a patient to expire after such a brief illness. The neurosurgeon stated that he could do nothing further for Mr. S, but that the decision to refuse further treatment was not his to make. The cardiologist was pleased with Mr. S's blood pressure reduction and his partial heart recovery and felt that he could not make a decision to discontinue treatment. The kidney specialist believed that dialysis might improve his general condition a little and could not take responsibility for any other course. The lung specialist could not make life-and-death decisions; his responsibility was the status of the patient's lungs, and they were doing well. The neurologist understood and agreed with Mrs. S but felt that his responsibility was only to evaluate the degree of damage. Mrs. S felt that no one was accepting responsibility for her husband's care.

> (Warren Point, 1999, personal communication)

One could conclude that since Mrs. S had made a request of the family physician, he should have assumed responsibility; or that since the neurosurgeon was listed as the attending physician, he should have dealt with the problem; or that the kidney specialist should have taken a more holistic approach and recommended against dialysis; or that the neurologist should have clearly indicated that Mr. S could not be saved and requested a medical team meeting. The problem was that no single member of this medical team took responsibility for making the decision to stop treatment. Cases like this can drag on without a solution until the patient dies—as happened in this instance. In the meantime, the lack of coordination and failure to assume responsibility can devastate patients and their families.

Initially, one would say that this is a clinical problem and requires a medical staff solution. The medical team needs to decide who is in charge. But if the medical team on a given case, or the medical staff as a whole, is unable or unwilling to address a problem, it becomes an administrative matter. Sooner or later, the administration may have to tell the medical staff that such situations are unacceptable. The administration may not have a responsibility to make clinical decisions, but it has a responsibility to see that such decisions are made.

MEDICAL RESEARCH: INSTITUTIONAL REVIEW BOARDS

The book, *Protecting Human Research Subjects: Institutional Review Board Guidebook*, published by the U.S. Department of Health and Human Services, perpetuates a commonly held belief:

> The modern story of human subjects protections begins with the Nuremberg Code, developed for the Nuremberg Military Tribunal as a standard by which to judge the human experimentation conducted by the Nazis.
>
> (OPPR, 1993: xviii)

The 1947 Nuremberg Code, however, is at best a symbolic beginning. The Code itself was formulated only *after* the trials as a reflection on the standards employed (Moreno, 1998). At the time, media attention to the Nazi atrocities was directed mostly to the incompetence and inhumanity of the experiments rather than to the use of human subjects without their consent: "The Nuremberg trial of the Nazi doctors . . . received very little press coverage, and before the 1970's, the code itself was infrequently cited or discussed in medical journals" (Rothman, 1995: 529). Throughout the 1950s, the U.S. military continued to conduct experiments on involuntary service personnel, and private sector medical research was continued without the informed consent of the subjects in the United States well into the 1970s (Beecher, 1966; Hastings, 1992). The Declaration of Helsinki was not adopted by the World Medical Association until 1964. The National Institutes of Health in the United States did not issue a policy on medical research until 1966, and this policy was not raised to regulatory status until 1974, when the Tuskegee Study was exposed (OPPR, 1993).

If the Nuremberg Code is now given too much credit, other developments are often given too little credit. In 1900 the Prussian government entirely prohibited medical intervention for purposes other than diagnosis, therapy, and immunization if a person was a minor or incompetent, and it prohibited experimentation on people who had not given fully informed consent (Capron, 1997). The U.S. Atomic Energy Commission had also considered the matter as early as 1947 and eventually developed a principle of informed consent, although its guidelines remained undisclosed for years (Moreno and Hurt, 1998).

The problem really came to the attention of the medical community in the United States in 1966 with the publication of Henry Beecher's article "Ethics and Clinical Research" in the *New England Journal of Medicine*. Beecher argued that "unethical or questionably ethical procedures are not uncommon" in medical research and cited 22 examples of studies in which the health of research subjects was endangered without informing them of the risk or obtaining their consent. Beecher determined that this research was not unusual; in fact, it was commonly sponsored by major universities and published in major biomedical journals. Patients in mental institutions were infected with malaria for the purpose of testing new drugs. Inmates of a youth correctional center were vaccinated against influenza A and B and then exposed to the virus, while the control group was injected with the virus alone. All of the studies cited by Beecher took place after 1950.

The public disclosure of the Tuskegee Study in 1972 elicited an even greater public response (Pence, 1995). Throughout the early decades of the twentieth century, American medicine and biology were demonstrably racist. African-Americans were commonly viewed as physically defective and mentally inferior, as well as emotionally uncontrollable. They were regarded by physicians and medical researchers alike as fit subjects for experimentation. Because earlier research on syphilis had raised questions about the effectiveness of the conventional treatment, it was considered important to chart the natural course of the disease in order to recognize significant changes. In the early 1930s the U.S. Public Health Service identified Macon County, Alabama, as one of six counties with exceptionally high rates of syphilis and initiated the study at the Tuskegee Institute. Its original purpose was to observe the progress of the disease in untreated African-American males. At the time, the available treatments appeared to relieve symptoms but not to control the disease. The study, which lasted from 1932 until 1972, was conducted in a haphazard manner. It had no director for much of that period, and visits from federal doctors were as infrequent as nine years apart. The 399 participants were deceived by being told that they had "bad blood" and that the spinal tap, which was done to measure the progress of the disease, was really a treatment. When penicillin became available between 1943 and 1945, none of the Tuskegee subjects were treated. This situation continued throughout the 1960s. In fact, some subjects were deferred from the draft during World War II because they would have received treatment in the army. As late as 1969 and with the subjects still untreated, a committee at the Centers for Disease Control voted to continue the study.

In 1972, Associated Press reporter Jean Heller wrote an article, "Syphilis Victims in U.S. Study Went Untreated for Forty Years," which appeared on the front page of the *New York Times*. The Tuskegee Study was closed later that year by the Secretary of Health and Human Services, and congressional hearings were held. The study had violated almost every rule of medical research now in effect. There was no informed consent, subjects were deceived, the presuppositions of the study were clearly racist, the research design was faulty, it produced no beneficial findings, and, above all, the participants were directly harmed.

In 1974, Congress passed the National Research Act establishing institutional review boards (IRBs) for research involving human subjects. A National Commission for the Protection of Human Subjects of Biomedical and Behavioral Research and its successor, the President's Commission for the Study of Ethical Problems in Medicine and Biomedical and Behavioral Research, issued reports on a wide range of problems in medical ethics. These reports, which generally upheld a strong patients' rights perspective, were influential in creating a national consensus on many bioethical issues.

The jurisdiction of IRBs expanded quickly from research undertaken by federal agencies, to research supported by federal funds, and then to all research at institutions receiving federal funds. Institutional review boards are institution specific, so a number of such boards may be operating in any given geographical area. Educational testing and survey research in which respondents are not identifiable are generally exempt from the review and consent process. Furthermore, IRB review covers only aspects of research that have to do with the protection of human subjects. Institutions may have other committees to judge the scientific value of research or to determine whether the institution will sponsor or permit the research. Standards developed by the JCAHO maintain that, in addition to IRB requirements for the protection of subjects, a hospital "always reviews research protocols in relation to the hospital's mission statement, values, and other guidelines" (JCAHO, 1996: RI-17).

Federal regulations specify the composition and jurisdiction of IRBs and the nature of their function in considerable detail (OPPR, 1993). Institutional Review Board approval for research with human subjects involves a number of ethical considerations. The first major issue is whether the research itself is justified by its potential benefit to individuals and to society in light of the risks involved. Here a distinction has to be made between research and therapy (although both are involved in many biomedical studies), and it is the specific risk associated with research that must be assessed. Patients may choose to accept other risks for therapeutic reasons. It is the task of the IRB to assess the risks associated with research and to weigh these risks against possible social benefits. Research risks may be physical or psychological, and an effort must be made to keep them to a minimum.

The second ethical consideration for IRB approval of a research protocol involves informed consent. Regulations here parallel those for consent to medical treatment generally, but with specific requirements that consent forms and explanations cover all issues related to the experimental nature of the drugs or procedures. Institutional review boards typically spend much of their time reviewing consent forms designed with local populations in mind. Research often involves placebos, randomization of subjects, and blind or double-masked protocols that have to be explained to subjects. Special situations involving deception or incomplete disclosure and the use of children or incapacitated adults as subjects must be considered very carefully.

The selection of appropriate subjects for research is a third ethical consideration. Initially there is the question of fairness. According to the Institutional Review Board *Guidebook*:

In the 19th and early 20th centuries, the burdens of research fell largely upon poor patients in hospital wards, while the benefits flowed primarily to private patients. This inequity was starkly revealed in the Tuskegee syphilis study, in which disadvantaged blacks in the rural south were recruited for studies of the untreated course of a disease that was by no means confined to that population. Such unjustified overutilization of certain segments of the population led the National Commission to recommend that selection of research subjects be scrutinized to determine "whether some classes (e.g., welfare patients, racial and ethnic minorities, or persons confined to institutions) are being systematically selected simply because of their easy availability, their compromised position or their manipulability, rather than for reasons directly related to the problem being studied."

(OPPR, 1993:3–23)

More recently, it is the compromised position of individuals, rather than their social class or race, that has made certain people appear to be more available as research subjects. Such persons include not only prisoners and patients in mental institutions, but also psychology students, medical students, military personnel, and employees of pharmaceutical companies who are in a compromised position because they are often dependent on superiors who may ask them to volunteer. Prison inmates who might volunteer if they are paid (and may have no other way of earning money) or who feel that they must appear cooperative to gain the favor of wardens or parole boards are especially vulnerable. They are also good subjects for research because they are generally healthy, and their diet and activity can be easily monitored. Although a great deal of drug research has been done with prisoners, many ethicists now argue that they cannot be considered uncompromised volunteers.

The historical exclusion of minorities and women from studies is also an issue. Institutional review board policy now requires the inclusion of women and minorities in research populations so that the findings, and eventual benefits, will be available to all people. Age is a more recent consideration. The exclusion of women, minorities, or the elderly, whether intentional or unintentional, can be discriminatory. If there are scientific reasons to anticipate differences among gender, racial, or age groups with regard to the treatment under investigation, the benefits of the study will not accrue to populations that are excluded. The IRB *Guidebook* includes a separate chapter on "Special Classes of Subjects" that focuses on women, minors, prisoners, cognitively impaired people, comatose and terminally ill people, minorities, the elderly, students, and employees.

A fourth ethical issue for IRB consideration is the confidentiality of research information. Since research information is collected and held in a manner different from that of other medical records, special care is needed. In particular, personal identifiers must be removed from records used in epidemiological studies, and the use of records for any purpose other than that for which they were collected without specific permission is morally unacceptable. Healthcare organizations should check IRB approval requirements as well as institutional policies very carefully before granting requests to review medical records for the purpose of identifying possible subjects. Until recently, it was common practice for research organizations and pharmaceutical companies to send agents to find subjects with certain medical conditions, and these agents were often permitted to review medical records at will in search of subjects. Information relating to sexual preferences or practices, drug or alcohol use, illegal conduct, and mental health, as well as information that might be of interest to employers or insurance companies, deserves special care in this context.

A practical risk associated with IRBs is that they may become captive to a medical research community that is more interested in publishable results than in the welfare of human subjects. Federal guidelines are designed to prevent this, but healthcare administrators responsible for research programs should also see to it that representatives of all stakeholder groups participate effectively in the review process.

Finally, it should be emphasized that the ethical responsibility of a healthcare organization with respect to medical research is not limited to the establishment of an IRB according to federal guidelines. From an ethical perspective, research should not only fulfill federal IRB requirements, it should also be consistent with the mission and goals of the healthcare organization. This is a matter of organizational ethics. If an IRB is not specifically charged with considering the conformity of medical research to organizational goals, a separate organizational review will be necessary.

Case 11.2 Disclosure of Payment

One current issue for many IRBs is whether all the financial aspects of research ought to be disclosed to potential subjects as part of the consent process. Let us suppose, for example, that a physician is asked to be a clinical investigator for a new drug. The composition of the drug is the proprietary property of a pharmaceutical company, but the field is competitive and other companies are rushing similar products to market. In addition to normal compensation for expenses, the manufacturer is offering the physician $600 per enrollee in the study and is willing to pay for expedited service and the additional time he will spend if he submits results within three months.

A member of one IRB asked to approve the study has pointed out that the Hospital Code of Ethics and the proposed federal Patients' Bill of Rights for Managed Care can be interpreted to require that all financial contingencies associated with clinical practice be disclosed to prospective subjects. The Hospital Ethics Code states that "all patients must be informed of any financial considerations that may affect their informed consent to treatment." The Patients' Bill of Rights for Managed Care states that "managed care plans are subject to full disclosure regarding benefits, access, out-of-area and emergency coverage, authorization and grievance procedures, utilization review and provider compensation."

The question before the IRB is whether the $600 paid to the physician should be disclosed to participants in the study. It is likely that some patients' decisions would be affected by this knowledge, but disclosure might also put research physicians in a bad light with a public that is already somewhat suspicious of medical research. The public, however, is ambivalent: on the one hand, many people distrust physicians when it comes to research; on the other hand, they want access to the latest experimental drugs. There is, furthermore, a question regarding the standard to be used in deciding what should be disclosed. Traditionally, only factors that involve an increased risk to patients must be disclosed. In this case, there is no added risk to subjects simply because they do not know about the financial arrangements between the physician and the pharmaceutical company. Some ethicists now argue, however, that the standard for disclosure should be whatever a patient might want to know and that some patients in this study might be interested in factors that might influence their physician's recommendations.

COMPLIANCE PROGRAMS

The major financial incentive for a hospital, nursing home, home health agency, or clinical laboratory to initiate a voluntary program to monitor compliance with federal law is that such programs reduce the risk of liability under Medicare and Medicaid regulations. The Office of the Inspector General (OIG), for example, will consider the existence of an effective compliance program that predated any governmental investigation when addressing the appropriateness of administrative penalties for violations of HCFA rules. The federal False Claims Act (31 U.S.C. §§ 3729–3733) provides that a person who has violated the act, but who voluntarily discloses the violation to the government, in certain circumstances will be subject to only double, as opposed to treble, damages.

The OIG *Compliance Program Guidelines* (OIG, 1998) document lists the following seven basic elements of a compliance program:

1. Written policies and procedures governing potential fraud.
2. The appointment of a compliance officer who reports directly to the governing board.
3. A compliance education program.
4. A complaint mechanism such as a hotline for reporting problems.
5. A system to respond to allegations of wrongdoing including disciplinary measures.
6. An ongoing audit program to monitor compliance.
7. A mechanism for corrective actions.

Many organizational programs have begun by appointing compliance officers, formulating codes of ethical conduct, developing educational programs, and establishing hotline response systems. Most have not yet developed systematic audit practices (see Chapter 12) or effective governing board involvement. A detailed account of these elements is given in the OIG *Guidelines*. The program is intended to cover abuses such as patients' lack of freedom of choice, billing for discharge instead of transfer, patient dumping, DRG inflation, and many other aspects of a healthcare organization's business operations.

Organizational–Professional Relations

One area of recent concern for compliance officers has been the business relationships that healthcare organizations have with professional providers and provider groups. The federal Anti-Kickback Statute (42 U.S.C. Section 1320a–7b(b)), which has been amended a number of times since its passage in 1972, and the Stark Legislation (42 U.S.C. Section 1395nn) of 1989 and 1993 have restructured in great detail the relationship between healthcare organizations and independent professional providers. The Anti-Kickback Statute prohibits remuneration of any kind for referring a Medicare or Medicaid patient to any provider or provider organization. A number of exemptions have been carved out, however, and *safe harbors* have been created. A safe harbor allows an offending party to escape prosecution by demonstrating that a practice was undertaken in the belief that it was legal and by repaying any funds received as a result of that practice.

Beginning in 1989, the OIG issued a number of "Fraud Alerts" interpreting the Anti-Kickback Statute. These Alerts cover joint ventures (1989), prescription drugs (1994), clinical laboratory services (1994), home health services (1995), and relations with nursing facilities (1995–1996). In its 1992 Fraud Alert on hospital incentives to physicians, for example, the OIG listed the following activities as potentially illegal:

1. Payment of any sort for referring a patient to a hospital
2. Provision of free or underpriced office space, equipment, or staff services
3. Free training in management techniques
4. Income guarantees
5. Low- or no-interest loans
6. Travel expenses
7. Continuing education fees
8. Free or low-priced insurance coverage
9. Payment for services not rendered or overvalued

The Stark Legislation further prohibits or limits physician referrals for health services to entities with which the physician has a financial relationship. Governmental oversight has become excessively complex. Regulations promulgated by the HCFA, OIG rules, and advisory opinions from the Secretary of Health and Human Services all specify guidelines that prohibit financial incentives. Even beyond the scope of the Anti-Kickback Statute and the Stark Legislation, the IRS is concerned that financial relationships may result in private gain from not-for-profit resources, thus endangering a healthcare organization's tax-exempt status. And since criminal prosecution is also mandated, the Justice Department is involved, and its interpretation of federal statutes and regulations may differ from that of other federal agencies.

Ethics and Compliance

Compliance programs are related to ethical concerns in a number of ways. First, inasmuch as ethical perspectives hold obedience to the law to be a moral obligation, compliance it itself an ethical value. Close attention to the spirit of the law, furthermore, can provide valuable guidance on many issues. Ethics goes beyond the law, of course, so compliance alone is not sufficient.

There is now considerable debate about the extent to which organizational ethics and compliance programs overlap. Both attempt to influence human behavior, and both involve norms or standards. Conceptual confusion may even be promoted by slogans like "Do It Right," which can be interpreted as either a legal or an ethical mandate. To a certain extent, however, the debate about the relationship between compliance and ethics is related to how compliance programs are understood. Compliance may be interpreted as simply legal compliance, or it may be interpreted as compliance with the law and with the goals of the organization. It is the source of the mandate, therefore, that marks the difference: for compliance, it is a civil code; for ethics, a philosophical imperative. This second understanding includes the ethical dimension as well as the legal one. In fact, the federal guidelines for organizational compliance programs mention ethical concerns as falling within the scope of compliance in this second sense:

> Fundamentally, compliance efforts are designed to establish a culture within a hospital that promotes prevention, detection and resolution of instances of conduct that do not conform to federal and state law, and federal, state and private payer health care program requirements, *as well as the hospital's ethical and business policies.* . . . It is incumbent upon a hospital's corporate officers and managers to provide ethical leadership to the organization and to assure that adequate systems are in place to facilitate *ethical and legal conduct.* Indeed, many hospitals and hospital organizations have adopted *mission statements articulating their commitment to high ethical standards.*
>
> (OIG, 1998; emphasis added)

Unfortunately, the federal guidelines do not expand on the concept of compliance with organizational ethics standards or mission goals. Beyond this brief note in the document's Introduction, there is no other mention of "ethical compliance," the ethical perspective, or the relationship between the two in the published guidelines. Most of the compliance literature and professional training, furthermore, exhibits an exclusively legal focus. The passage quoted above does, however, provide an indication of an important distinction. A compliance program can, if the organization chooses, include the notion of compliance with organizational goals and ethical principles in addition to regulatory compliance. This would give the program a dual focus, however, and it would be important for the program to be conceived as having a double obligation. If compliance is understood to include compliance with an organization's code of conduct and consistency with its mission statement, then the mandate of a compliance office would cover organizational ethics as well as legal compliance. If not, compliance would remain strictly legal in nature.

There is considerable overlap between organizational ethics and legal compliance, just as there is overlap between clinical ethics and laws regarding informed consent, resuscitation, and surrogate decision making. This overlap is perhaps most evident at a functional level. Both initiatives have an oversight responsibility, and both seek to influence people's work behavior. There are a number of common tasks, like detecting and addressing activities, that need to be corrected. It would make little sense for an organization to have one hotline for people to report legal compliance concerns and another for ethical concerns—a legal concern that funds are being diverted, for example, as opposed to an ethical concern that organizational resources are simply being wasted. There are also, of course, distinct differences. Just as legal regulations do not dictate ethical decisions in the clinical realm, compliance guidelines do not dictate the whole of an organization's mission statement or ethical standards; in fact, they specify very little of it.

The ethical mandate of a compliance program, therefore, is a matter for organizational decisions. If compliance is defined as compliance with the mission and values of the organization as well as compliance with the law, organizational ethics would fall within the purview of a compliance program. If compliance with the goals of an organization is not addressed by the compliance office, however, a separate organizational ethics program would be needed.

CONCLUSIONS

Clinical medical ethics committees, IRBs, and compliance programs all have responsibilities that extend into the domain of organizational ethics. As organizational groups, they have obligations to the goals of the institution. Clinical ethics committees focus on problems of patient care, but the coordination of that care within institutional policies and procedures is an administrative matter as well. Institutional review boards have specific ethical responsibilities under federal law, but they also have a responsibility to consider whether research is appropriate in light of the organization's goals. Compliance programs audit activities for consistency with federal and state regulations, but they may also (if institutions so choose) audit activities for consistency with organizational mission statements and ethical guidelines. Administrators have a responsibility to see that these programs advance the goals of the institution and that they are carried out with consideration of the interests of all who have a stake in their activities.

REFERENCES

Arras, John D., and Bonnie Steinbock, eds., 1999, *Ethical Issues in Modern Medicine*, 5th ed., Mountain View, CA: Mayfield Publishing Company.

ASBH (American Society for Bioethics and Humanities), 1998, *Core Competencies for Health Care Ethics Consultation*, Glenville, IL: American Society for Bioethics and Humanities.

Beauchamp, Tom L., and James F. Childress, 1994, *Principles of* Biomedical *Ethics*, 4th ed., New York: Oxford University Press.

Beauchamp, Tom L., and Leroy Walters, eds., 1999, *Contemporary Issues in Bioethics*, 4th ed., Belmont, CA: Wadsworth Publishing Company.

Beecher, Henry E., 1966, "Ethics and Clinical Research," *New England Journal of Medicine*, 274:1354–1360.

Capron, A. M., 1997, "Human Experimentation," in Robert M. Veatch, ed., *Medical Ethics*, 2nd ed., Boston: Jones and Bartlett Publishers.

Christensen, Kate T., and Robin Tucker, 1997, "Ethics without Walls: The Transformation of Ethics Committees in the New Healthcare Environment," *Cambridge Quarterly of Healthcare Ethics*, 6:299–301.

De Vries, Raymond, and Janardan Subedi, eds., 1998, *Bioethics and Society*, Upper Saddle River, NJ: Prentice-Hall.

Fletcher, Joseph F., 1955, *Morals and Medicine*, London: Victor Gollancz Limited.

Hastings (The Hastings Center), 1987, *Guidelines on the Termination of Life-Sustaining Treatment and the Care of the Dying*, Bloomington, IN: Indiana University Press.

————, 1992, "Twenty Years After: The Legacy of the Tuskegee Syphilis Study," *Hastings Center Report*, 22:29–40.

Heller, Jean, 1972, "Syphilis Victims in U.S. Study Went Untreated for Forty Years," *New York Times*, July 26, A1.

JCAHO (Joint Commission on Accreditation of Healthcare Organizations), 1996, *Comprehensive Accreditation Manual for Hospitals: The Official Handbook. Refreshed Core, January 1998*, Oakbrook Terrace, IL: Joint Commission on Accreditation of Healthcare Organizations.

Lo, Bernard, 1996, *Resolving Ethical Dilemmas: A Guide for Clinicians*, Baltimore: Williams and Wilkins.

Moreno, Jonathan D., 1998, "The Pentagon Meets the Nuremberg Code: A Study in Organizational Ethics," paper presented at the conference "A New National Agenda: Organizational Ethics in Health Care," Olsson Center for Applied Ethics, University of Virginia, September 25.

Moreno, Jonathan D., and Valerie Hurt, 1998, "How the Atomic Energy Commission Discovered 'Informed Consent'," in Raymond DeVries and Janardan Subedi, eds., *Bioethics and Society*, Upper Saddle River, NJ: Prentice-Hall.

OIG (Office of the Inspector General of the Department of Health and Human Services), 1998, "The Office of the Inspector General's Compliance Program Guidance for Hospitals," http://www.dhhs.gov/progorg/oig/modcomp/index.htm (10/25/98).

OPPR (Office for Protection from Research Risks, National Institutes of Health, United States Department of Health and Human Services), 1993, *Protecting Human Research Subjects: Institutional Review Board Guidebook*, Washington, DC: U.S. Government Printing Office.

Pence, Gregory E., 1995, *Classic Cases in Medical Ethics*, 2nd ed., New York: McGraw-Hill.

Ramsey, Paul, 1970, *The Patient as Person*, New Haven, CT: Yale University Press.

Rothman, David J., 1995, "Ethics and Human Experimentation: Henry Beecher Revisited," in John D. Arras and Bonnie Steinbock, eds., *Ethical Issues in Modern Medicine*, 4th ed., Mountain View, CA: Mayfield Publishing Company.

Thomas, Clayton L., ed., 1993, *Taber's Cyclopedic Medical Dictionary*, 17th ed., Philadelphia: F. A. Davis Company.

Thomasma, David C., and Thomasine Kushner, 1996, *Birth to Death: Science and Bioethics*, Cambridge, UK: Cambridge University Press.

Veatch, Robert M., ed., 1997, *Medical Ethics*, 2nd ed., Sudbury, MA: Jones and Bartlett Publishers.

Wolf, Susan M., ed., 1996, *Feminism and Bioethics: Beyond Reproduction*, New York: Oxford University Press.

12

THE DEVELOPMENT OF AN ORGANIZATIONAL ETHICS PROGRAM

The current move toward healthcare organizational ethics involves both carrots and sticks. The carrots are the desires of many healthcare professionals to build a better healthcare system. These people take seriously the unmet needs of those who have no health insurance, the social responsibilities of businesses, the community obligations of nonprofit organizations, and the organizational problems of institutions. The sticks are the patients' rights movement in managed care, compliance with federal regulations, and the standards set by the JCAHO. This chapter reviews the JCAHO'S standards, discusses options for establishing an organizational ethics program, and proposes two practical strategies for program implementation.

THE STANDARDS OF THE JOINT COMMISSION ON ACCREDITATION OF HEALTHCARE ORGANIZATIONS

Since 1995 JCAHO has included organizational ethics in its standards on patient rights (JCAHO 1996:RI–4). *Standards*, in JCAHO terminology, refer to general goals. The practice of the Commission is to set goals and to expect that healthcare institutions will fulfill these goals in different ways. The standards, therefore, do not have much detail.

Under the section entitled "Patients Rights and Organizational Ethics," JCAHO standards address four general topics: ethical issues in patient care (RI.1), organ procurement and donation policy (RI.2), medical research involving human subjects (RI.3), and the organizational code of ethical behavior (RI.4) (JCAHO, 1998a). The first three generally fall within the scope of organizational committees. Medical ethics is covered by clinical committees, organ procurement and donation is often assigned to a special interdisciplinary committee, and patients' rights in clinical research fall under the jurisdiction of IRBs governed by federal regulations. The JCAHO organizational ethics standards are as follows:

> RI.4 The hospital operates according to a code of ethical behavior.
> RI.4.1 The code addresses marketing, admission, transfer and discharge, and billing practices.
> RI.4.2 The code addresses the relationship of the hospital and its staff members to other health care providers, educational institutions and payers.
> RI.4.3 In hospitals with longer lengths of stay, the code addresses a patient's rights to perform or refuse to perform tasks in or for the hospital.
> RI.4.4 The hospital's code of ethical business and professional behavior protects the integrity of clinical decision making, regardless of how the hospital compensates or shares financial risk with its leaders, managers, clinical staff, and licensed independent practitioners.
>
> (JCAHO, 1998a:55–56)

Standards RI.4.2 and RI.4.4 are further explained in the following Intent statements:

Intent of RI.4 Through RI.4.2

A hospital has an ethical responsibility to the patients and community it serves. Guiding documents such as the hospital's mission statement and strategic plan, provide a consistent, ethical framework for its patient care and business practices. But a framework alone is not sufficient. To support ethical operations and fair treatment of patients, a hospital has and operates according to a code of ethical behavior. The code addresses ethical practices regarding marketing, admission, transfer, discharge, billing, and resolution of conflicts associated with patient billing. The code ensures that the hospital conducts its business and patient care practices in an honest, decent and proper manner.

(JCAHO, 1998a:55)

Intent of RI.4.4

To avoid compromising the quality of care, clinical decisions (including tests, treatments, and other interventions) are based on identified patient health care needs. The hospital's code of ethical business and professional behavior specifies that the hospital implements policies and procedures that address the relationship between the use of services and financial incentives. Policies and procedures addressing information on this issue are available on request to all patients, clinical staff, licensed independent practitioners and hospital personnel.

(JCAHO, 1998a:56)

The larger JCAHO *Comprehensive Accreditation Manual for Hospitals* (JCAHO, 1996) includes various examples and practical applications, but the substance is contained in the Standards and Intent statements quoted here. The JCAHO also offers a number of considerations relevant to its standards and the development of organizational ethics programs in its publication *Ethical Issues and Patient Rights Across the Continuum of Care* (1998b). This book includes a helpful list of topics that an organizational ethics program should address which is reprinted in Appendix 6.

The JCAHO views organizational ethics in terms of an institutional code that assures patients appropriate service with regard to the business arrangements of their health care. Its major focus here is clearly on patients' rights, as indicated in this introductory paragraph of its Overview:

The goal of the patients rights and organization ethics function is to help improve patient outcomes by respecting each patient's rights and conducting business relationships with patients and the public in an ethical manner.

(JCAHO, 1998a:45)

This focus, however, somewhat limits the scope of the JCAHO's ethical considerations. Other people who have an important stake in business decisions made by healthcare institutions are given only brief mention in these standards. Fair evaluation practices, reasonable privacy, occupational safety, and protection for whistle-blowing are important for employees. Use of competitive bidding, trust in contract negotiations and restrictions on gratuities are important to suppliers and other business partners. Compliance with public health, zoning, tax, and other government regulations is important to the public interest; employment opportunities and environmental protection are important to the surrounding community. The JCAHO standards indicate that hospitals have responsibilities to the communities they serve, but the service area may or may not be the same as the community in which the hospital is located. For example, a hospital may serve only veterans or people with specific illnesses, and thus may not serve all or even most of the people in the community where it is located. Thus there are a number of organizational ethics questions, many of which have been discussed in the preceding chapters, that are not related primarily to patients' rights and are therefore omitted from JCAHO consideration. It can be expected that these issues will come more into focus as the JCAHO standards evolve in future years.

MODELS FOR ORGANIZATIONAL ETHICS PROGRAMS

In light of the JCAHO standards, healthcare organizations are now required to develop organizational ethics programs (Khushf, 1997). There are five possible models for such programs. These models are not mutually exclusive alternatives, but they differ in strategy and emphasis.

The Existing Hospital Ethics Committee

If a healthcare organization has an ethics committee that deals with clinical matters, the scope of this committee could be expanded to cover organizational ethics (Thompson, 1992; Weber, 1997). There are advantages to this approach, but there are also serious disadvantages. If a hospital ethics committee handles the traditional tasks of consultation, policy development, and education, for example, expanding its scope to organizational ethics may be difficult. First, if the committee is active, it may already have enough to do without taking on what is, in effect, a different field. Second, the committee may not have members from the organizational management side of the institution, so it would have to be expanded (ASBH, 1998). Even then, the impression might prevail within the organization that a patient care committee is meddling in business decisions. Third, organizational ethics issues are significantly different from clinical issues, and it is reasonable to ask whether the members of existing medical ethics committees have the educational background or skills to deal with these problems. A report titled *Core Competencies for Health Care Ethics Consultation*, published by the American Society for Bioethics and Humanities, establishes serious educational requirements for patient consultation (ASBH, 1998); it would seem reasonable for people dealing with organizational ethics to have comparable backgrounds—MBA, MPH, or MHA degrees, along with training in law, economics, and business ethics. If the task of organizational ethics is to be assigned to the existing clinical ethics committee, one would have to consider the membership and professional expertise of the participants (Schneider-O'Connell, 1995).

On the other hand, an advantage to this model is that an existing ethics committee may have a recognized position in a healthcare organization from which certain organizational ethics issues can be addressed effectively (Thompson, 1992). It may have the respect of both administrative and direct provider professionals that will facilitate the handling of these new issues. It may have an existing mode of operation with lines of education and communication that will promote organizational development (ASBH, 1998). Dr. Edward Spencer (1997) of the University of Virginia has made a strong case to the effect that hospital ethics committees should adopt this new organizational role. Still, as William Atchley (1992:212) has said, "it remains to be seen whether the ethics committee is the best forum for establishing institutional and social policy." There is a great difference between organizational ethics issues, as discussed above, and the normal concerns of clinical ethics committees. According to the JCAHO, "In larger or more complex health care organizations, such as tertiary care centers, maintaining two distinct functions— clinical ethics and organizational ethics—might be the most effective approach, owing to the often complicated nature of the issues that these organizations face" (JCAHO, 1998b:69). In any case, assigning responsibility for organizational ethics to an existing clinical ethics committee is not a step that should be taken lightly.

An Ethics Officer or Consultant

A second option is the appointment of an organizational ethics officer or consultant. This is not uncommon in major corporations, where ethics officers usually fit into organizational structures in strategic planning, risk management, compliance, or legal divisions (Hoffman, 1995). Since ethical considerations have to be dealt with at the top of the organizational structure, however, it is important for an ethics officer to be able to communicate directly with top management and the governing board.

The major advantage of an ethics officer is that there is someone in the organization who is specifically assigned to look at organizational activities from an ethical perspective. With committees or administrators with a whole raft of other duties, it may be all too easy to ignore the ethical dimension. The major disadvantage of this model is that ethical considerations that should become a regular dimension of managerial decision making may be left entirely to the ethics officer. The ethics officer may then become marginalized within the organizational structure as an informal way of avoiding controversial issues.

Ethics and Compliance

In many respects, the most logical place for an organizational ethics program is within a compliance office. Functionally, there is great similarity here; a compliance program must secure compliance with the mandates of state and federal laws, while an ethics program aims to bring about compliance with the organization's code of conduct and mission statement. Both are oversight functions that reach into every aspect of an organization's activity. There are aspects of ethical concern, such as community relations and corporate social responsibility, that lie outside the concern of the law, but there are many more issues in which overlap is unavoidable. The federal OIG, as mentioned earlier, has included ethical considerations within the scope of its guidelines for compliance programs.

One clear advantage of placing an ethics program in a compliance office is the consolidation of functions. Both programs need some mechanism by which people can report concerns—a telephone hotline or an officer who will investigate a problem. Another advantage of an ethics program attached to a compliance office is that the compliance office, according to federal guidelines, has direct access to the governing board. A third possible advantage is that this structure sends a clear message throughout the organization that adherence to ethical standards is as important as legal compliance.

An obvious disadvantage of this model is that the compliance program may have too much of a legal orientation. This arrangement might be understood to imply that if an action is legal, it is ethically acceptable. Much depends on how the mandate of a compliance program is framed. If compliance is viewed primarily as regulatory compliance, the concept of organizational ethics will have a difficult time gaining a proper foothold.

Governing Board Committee

A fourth alternative is the appointment of a subcommittee of the governing board with responsibility for meeting with management and reporting back to the board on a regular basis. This clearly places ethical considerations at an organizational level where they can be most influential. It is widely accepted in business ethics that unless there is a commitment to ethical practices at the top, the corporate culture is unlikely to pay much attention to the ethical dimension. According to Donna J. Wood of the University of Pittsburgh's Joseph M. Katz Graduate School of Business, "Virtually every writer who addresses the subject of institutionalizing business ethics emphasizes one crucial factor: the commitment of senior management, and particularly the chief executive officer" (Wood, 1990:254).

The downside of this model is that the ethical issues handled by the governing board may be so generalized that the ethics program will not reach into the details of day-to-day operations. The program may thus become marginalized by being considered too important to address lower-level decisions. Ethical issues need to be addressed not only as they arise, but before they arise. An organizational structure that addresses ethical issues only when they have become problematic enough to merit governing board attention will miss many opportunities.

Management Discussion Group

A final model for organizational ethics programs is the creation of a high-level management discussion group. Discussion groups are more advisory (to those who bring up the issues for discussion and must eventually make the decisions) than authoritative. An informal discussion group can be an effective means of enhancing trust among major decision makers and a way of listening to people who have a stake in organizational decisions if they are represented in the discussion. But a discussion group designed for the informal exchange of ideas may also lack the authority to make its influence felt. So while this approach may foster a corporate culture in which ethical issues are discussed more freely, it may not have much actual effect on organizational policy or practice. Administrators would be free to avoid submitting issues for discussion and to ignore the advice offered. To be realistic, those who are most in need of ethics advice may opt out of the process.

The models mentioned here clearly each have pros and cons, and different approaches will be effective at different institutions. As noted above, these approaches are not mutually exclusive: one could have an ethics officer with a board committee, a compliance program, or a management discussion group. Although a combination of approaches could be adopted since each has unique benefits, the resulting duplication might not be desirable. The development of an effective program depends to a very large extent on the nature of the organization.

Whatever model or combination of models is chosen, two factors are significant. The first is support from top management (Hofmann, 1994). As James Sabin and Lisa Raiola (1998:30) put it: "If the CEO does not regard himself as the 'Chief Ethics Officer' it is probably unwise to develop a formal program" (see also Hofmann, 1994). The second factor is the openness and representativeness of the process. An effective organizational ethics program needs to be open to issues that arise at every level within the organization and to issues that arise outside the organizational structure—from patients, the community, suppliers, and healthcare professionals. The decision-making process, furthermore, needs to include the ethical perspectives of all who will be affected by organizational actions. This can be accomplished in various ways, ranging from a process in which those giving the ethical advice attempt to consider the consequences of their actions for the people involved to a participatory process that actually brings representative stakeholders to the table.

FROM ETHICAL PERSPECTIVES TO OPERATIONAL STRATEGIES

While there is more to be said about the development of organizational ethics programs, most decisions in this area will be institution-specific. Rather than elaborate the alternatives, it will be more helpful here to shift our focus to the ways in which an organizational ethics program might function. Two operational strategies can be used to carry ethical analysis forward in a systematic manner.

The Advisory Opinion Strategy

The first strategy is a process for advisory opinions. State governments have had considerable success with the process of submitting individual managerial decisions to state ethics commissions for advance approval or an advisory opinion. Ethical dilemmas are rarely matters of clear right and wrong. Public officials, like healthcare managers, are often in doubt as to whether a proposed course of action is ethically acceptable. The advisory opinion process gives public employees a way to have decisions reviewed and advice proffered before actions are taken. It can also assure administrators that if they follow the advice, their actions will not later be found to have violated state governmental ethics laws. In state government this has led to the accumulation of a sizable body of decisions that serve as precedents for future actions. The ethical dimension of public activity thus becomes a normal part of official decision making (Hall, 1989). Questions that arise later can be reviewed in the light of previous advisory opinions and expanded or adapted as necessary. The system has the great advantage of getting questions raised, discussed, and answered before decisions are made.

The same process could work well for a healthcare organizational ethics program. By submitting proposed decisions for review, managers can obtain advice that can be incorporated later into their decision making. This process clearly has much in common with the case consultation process currently in use by clinical ethics committees. For the most part, clinical ethics consultations are advisory to patients and physicians. The difference is that an institutional advisory opinion process builds up a set of organizational guidelines that can be made available for reference by others in similar situations. This works well for issues like conflicts of interest, where problematic situations are likely to recur, although there will also be cases with unique characteristics or circumstances.

Consider, for example, a simple question of travel expenses. A public relations manager is traveling across the country to attend a conference. When the conference is over, she wants to stay an extra week to visit her sister. Can she delay her return flight (paid for by the medical center) to make a personal visit? The organizational ethics committee says "Yes" as long as *(1)* the trip itself is approved as necessary for organizational purposes, *(2)* the annual leave is approved for that time period, and *(3)* both approvals come from a higher level. This opinion would then set a precedent for anyone in a similar situation in the future, and employees could rest assured that if they follow the rules, no ethical issues will be raised.

The major difficulty with this operational strategy is that important issues may not be submitted for consideration. People who are involved in questionable actions have interest in keeping those actions from coming to the attention of others. Some issues, furthermore, may be considered too confidential to be brought to committee meetings. This can be especially true if an organizational ethics committee is so constructed as to involve employee, community, or public stakeholders. So the committee may also need a separate process for dealing with requests confidentially.

Submitting an issue to an organizational ethics committee for consideration requires a certain amount of trust on the part of the person making the submission. Those who are asked to consider the problem may not sense the same pressures or tensions as the person whose decision is at issue. Sometimes people fear that they will be perceived as incompetent if they ask advice (a stereotypically male characteristic in our society); at other times, people may fear that others will consider their reservations about decisions to be trivial (a stereotypically female characteristic). The effectiveness of ethics case discussions depends on the establishment of trust within the ethics program.

Developing effective ethics discussions is not easy: in work situations people do not normally speak in terms of decisions being ethical or unethical, or morally right or wrong. These are loaded terms, and raising ethical questions can seem uncooperative or even accusatory. But issues need not be designated ethical to be considered from an ethical perspective: people often speak of being comfortable or uncomfortable with certain decisions and actions. The language isn't as important as the substance: if administrators want to consider ethical questions as only the social or public aspects of issues, fine. If administrators analyze the corporate culture or public relations dimensions of administrative decisions (i.e., how the alternatives affect the culture or image of the organization), this can cover a lot of ethical ground.

The Social Audit

The second operational strategy for organizational ethics programs is the social audit. In recent years, both academic researchers and corporate executives have been using the social audit to assess the relationship between organizations and their stakeholders (Wood, 1990; Zedek et al., 1997). Social auditing is a procedure for tracking the ethical performance of an organization. The Body Shop International, a major producer of cosmetics and health products, and the American ice cream company Ben and Jerry's Homemade, Inc., have undertaken extensive social audits and published their results since the early 1990s. Research organizations such as the New Economics Foundation (NEF, 1998a), Traidcraft Exchange (Traidcraft, 1998), and the Centre for Social and Environmental Accounting Research (CSEAR, 1999) have developed social accounting models and systems and serve as external auditors.

While the implementation of a social audit can be as extensive as one wishes to make it, the basic idea is relatively simple. Just as a financial audit gathers information, summarizes activities, uses standards to assess performance, and publishes a report to shareholders, a social audit collects information, develops assessment standards, and publishes a report on the social impact of an organization. The audit can involve considerable planning, including the identification of stakeholder relationships and interests, consultation with stakeholder groups, clarification of organizational values and goals, and an analytical feedback process. The Body Shop "Values Report 1997" runs to 208 pages plus an additional 40 pages of methodology (The Body Shop, 1998). This is clearly too elaborate for a fledgling healthcare organizational ethics program, but the extensive literature on social auditing provides a wealth of ideas and directions for consideration.

Many hospitals already publish annual reports listing levels of charitable care and community programs; some report patient satisfaction, employee satisfaction, and other indicators of social performance. A systematic audit procedure would regularize this process by establishing goals and tracking progress. Social factors can be as important to the success of an institution in carrying out its mission as financial statements can be to its solvency or stability. Yet social goals are seldom given as careful scrutiny as financial objectives. Periodic review of social progress by administrators and governing boards through the social audit can put both the mission of an institution and its important stakeholder relationships on the agendas of organizations in a new way.

Simon Zadek of the New Economics Foundation and his colleagues (Zadek et al., 1997) have listed eight principles of a social audit. These can be applied to healthcare organizations as follows.

1. *Inclusivity.* The social audit should be made from the perspectives of all stakeholders, not just that of the stockholders, governing board, or top managers. Assessment must involve not only how organizational activities affect stakeholders, but also how stakeholders themselves evaluate those activities.

2. *Comparability.* A basis of comparison has to be established for any social audit. This can involve both the historical performance of the organization itself (an annual accounting that will show progress or shortcomings) and external benchmarks when those are available. Examples of benchmarks might be the number of people served by the organization's public programs or the comparison of employees' wages with regional data.

3. *Completeness.* "The principle of completeness," according to Zadek et al. (1997:42), "means that no area of the company's activities can be deliberately and systematically excluded from the assessment." This principle is important to ensure that the organization does not use the audit merely to highlight its successes or ignore its failures.

4. *Evolution.* It should be expected that a social audit program may not cover all organizational activities the first year. Social auditing is conceived as an evolving and progressive activity.

5. *Management systems.* Management policies and systems are involved in the social audit process to the extent that some record keeping is necessary for the activity to be effective. Without systematic and accurate data collection on services, no audit is possible.

6. *Disclosure.* Social audits can be conducted either as an internal management tool or as an exercise in public accountability. The latter is clearly preferred, although most organizations would not want to engage in a public process before they knew what the consequences might be. Public accountability, however, is the ultimate objective of social responsibility.

7. *External verification.* A goal of the social audit process is to employ as much external verification in the process as is applied to financial audits. This is difficult to do at the moment because the process of social auditing is in its infancy and external experts are not generally available; this principle establishes a high ideal.

8. *Continuous improvement.* The ultimate objective of any social audit program is to assess progress. In ethics, as in any other aspect of organizational management, the establishment of goals and objectives that reflect an organization's values and the maintenance of a trajectory toward those goals and objectives is the key to success. Social performance, like efficiency, productivity, and customer satisfaction, is a matter of continued improvement (Carmichael et al., 1998).

Again, the detailed application of all these principles could be an overwhelming task. Corporations like Ben and Jerry's and The Body Shop that undertake social auditing have programs that have evolved over a number of years. The list of principles presented by Zadek et al. (1997) can serve as a way of illustrating the process and as a benchmark for the development of an organizational ethics program. An introductory version of a social audit for a healthcare organization would aim at assessing the major social effects of organizational activities for the major stakeholder groups. Points that might be addressed include patient satisfaction, investigation of complaints, transfer and discharge records, billing accuracy, employee complaints, employee training and advancement, uncompensated care, community health programs, and environmental issues.

A new organizational program should not be expected to address an extensive list of issues. It is better to focus on areas that can be covered well than to be too ambitious at the outset. The process, however, can provide an operational strategy to assist an organizational ethics program in getting on with the task. A program could begin simply by conducting an audit of employee and customer attitudes and build from there (NEF, 1998b).

Morality, as I mentioned at the outset, is a matter both of ideals to which one is attracted and social norms with sanctions. Social audit procedures focus primarily on the ideals—the goals to strive for. A natural sequel to the social audit, however, is to offer rewards for fulfilling organizational goals. This can be done in terms of employee evaluation. If employees are rewarded for meeting ethical goals as well as for meeting financial goals, the ethical performance of the organization will come to have as much significance as the financial performance. Allied Chemical reported a dramatic decrease in workplace accidents when it began to evaluate managers on their safety end environmental records as well as on the usual productivity measures (Metzger et al., 1993). It is naive, according to D. R. Cressey and C. A. Moore (1983), to believe that stern statements about the importance of ethical conduct alone will have much effect. Ethical behavior should be rewarded and tracked, and the rewards themselves can become a part of the ethical audit. Otherwise, according to Michael Metzger and colleagues (1993), reward systems are often counterproductive, reinforcing behavior that entirely misses the stated goals of the organization.

CONCLUSIONS

One conclusion from this discussion is that organizational ethics should not be considered merely an extension of medical ethics that can be left to existing clinical ethics committees without modification of membership and procedures. The issues are different, the players are different, the required skills and experience are different, and the goals are different. Models for the establishment of organizational ethics programs include redesigning existing ethics committees, appointing an institutional ethics officer, expanding a compliance program, assigning oversight to a subcommittee of the governing board, or convening a representative discussion group. Even if an organizational ethics program is avowedly pluralistic in its ethical perspectives, it will nonetheless be necessary to settle on an operational strategy for addressing the issues involved. Two strategies are suggested here. The advisory opinion model drawn from the experience of governmental ethics programs can lead to the development of a body of decisions that may influence the culture of an organization. The social audit process can bring ethical issues up for review by senior management and governing boards on a regular basis.

REFERENCES

ASBH (American Society for Bioethics and Humanities), 1998, *Core Competencies for Health Care Ethics Consultation*, Glenville, IL: American Society for Bioethics and Humanities.
Atchley, William A., 1992, "Commentary," *Cambridge Quarterly of Healthcare Ethics*, 1(3):212–213.

Carmichael, Sheena, Harry Hummels, Arco ten Klooster, and Henk van Luijk, 1998, *How Ethical Auditing Can Help Companies Compete More Effectively at an International Level*, Breukelen, the Netherlands: European Institute for Business Ethics.

Cressey, D. R., and C. A. Moore, 1983, "Managerial Values and Corporate Codes of Ethics," *California Management Review*, 25(4):53–57.

CSEAR (Centre for Social and Environmental Accounting Research), 1999, "Center for Social and Environmental Accounting Research," http://www.dundee.ac.uk/accountancy/csear/ (4/3/99).

Hall, Robert T., 1989, *The West Virginia Governmental Ethics Act: Text and Commentary*, Charleston, WV: Mountain State Press.

Hoffman, W. Michael, 1995, "A Blueprint for Corporate Ethical Development," in W. Michael Hoffman and Robert E. Frederick, eds., *Business Ethics: Readings and Cases in Corporate Morality*, 3rd ed., New York: McGraw-Hill.

Hofmann, Paul B., 1994, "Creating an Organizational Conscience: Ultimately, It Is the CEO's Responsibility to Establish the Moral Tone of the Organization," *Healthcare Executive*, 9(6):43–48.

JCAHO (Joint Commission on Accreditation of Healthcare Organizations), 1996, *Comprehensive Accreditation Manual for Hospitals: The Official Handbook. Update, May, 1997*, Oakbrook Terrace,IL: Joint Commission on Accreditation of Healthcare Organizations.

——, 1998a, *HAS: 1998 Hospital Accreditation Standards*, Oakbrook Terrace, IL: Joint Commission on Accreditation of Healthcare Organizations.

——, 1998b, *Ethical Issues and Patient Rights Across the Continuum of Care*, Oakbrook Terrace, IL: Joint Commission on Accreditation of Healthcare Organizations.

Khushf, George, 1997, "Administrative and Organizational Ethics," *HealthCare Ethics Committee Forum*, 9(4):299–309.

Metzger, Michael, Dan R. Dalton, and John W. Hill, 1993, "The Organization of Ethics and the Ethics of Organizations: The Case for Expanded Organizational Ethics Audits," *Business Ethics Quarterly*, 3(1):27–43.

NEF (New Economics Foundation), 1998a, "New Economics Foundation," http://sosig.ac.uk/NewEconomics/newecon.html (11/12/98).

——, 1998b, *Social Auditing for Small Organizations*, London: New Economics Foundation.

Sabin, James E., and Lee Raiola, 1998, "Four Reasons Not to Create an Ethics Program and Two Reasons to Do It," *Group Practice Journal*, February, 30–32.

Schneider-O'Connell, A., 1995. "A Corporate Ethics Committee in the Making," *HealthCare Ethics Committee Forum*, 7(4):264–272.

Spencer, Edward M., 1997, "A New Role for Institutional Ethics Committees: Organizational Ethics," *The Journal of Clinical Ethics*, 8(4):372–376.

The Body Shop, 1998, "Values Report 1997," http://www.the-body-shop.com (11/12/98).

Thompson, Dennis F., 1992, "Hospital Ethics," *Cambridge Quarterly of Healthcare Ethics*, 1(3):203–210.

Traidcraft, 1998, "Social Accounting," http://www.globalnet.co.uk/~traidcraft/sasumm.html (11/12/98); and http://www.traidcraft.co.uk/ (11/12/98).

Weber, Leonard J., 1997, "Taking on Organizational Ethics," *Health Progress,* 78(3):20–23.

Wood, Donna J., 1990, *Business and Society*, New York: HarperCollins Publishers.

Zadek, Simon, Peter Pruzan, and Richard Evans, eds., 1997, *Building Corporate Accountability: Emerging Practice in Social and Ethical Accounting, Auditing and Reporting*, London: New Economics Foundation.

Appendix 1

American Hospital Association

Management Advisory: Ethical Conduct for Health Care Institutions

INTRODUCTION

Health care institutions,* by virtue of their roles as health care providers, employers, and community health resources, have special responsibilities for ethical conduct and ethical practices that go beyond meeting minimum legal and regulatory standards. Their broad range of patient care, education, public health, social service, and business functions is essential to the health and well being of their communities. These roles and functions demand that health care organizations conduct themselves in an ethical manner that emphasizes a basic community service orientation and justifies the public trust. The health care institution's mission and values should be embodied in all its programs, services, and activities.

Because health care organizations must frequently seek a balance among the interests and values of individuals, the institution, and society, they often face ethical dilemmas in meeting the needs of their patients and their communities.

---

*The term *health care institution* represents the mission, programs, and services as defined and implemented by the institution's leadership, including the governing board, executive management, and medical staff leadership.

http://www.aha.org/resource/hethics.html (12/12/99). Reprinted with permission of the American Hospital Association, copyright 1999.

This advisory is intended to assist members of the American Hospital Association to better identify and understand the ethical aspects and implications of institution policies and practices. It is offered with the understanding that each institution's leadership in making policy and decisions must take into account the needs and values of the institution, its physicians, other caregivers, and employees and those of individual patients, their families, and the community as a whole.

The governing board of the institution is responsible for establishing and periodically evaluating the ethical standards that guide institutional policies and practices. The governing board must also assure that its own policies, practices, and members comply with both legal and ethical standards of behavior. The chief executive officer is responsible for assuring that hospital medical staff, employees, and volunteers and auxilians understand and adhere to these standards and for promoting a hospital environment sensitive to differing values and conducive to ethical behavior.

This advisory examines the hospital's ethical responsibilities to its community and patients as well as those deriving from its organizational roles as employer and business entity. Although explicit responsibilities also are included in legal and accreditation requirements, it should be remembered that legal, accreditation, and ethical obligations often overlap and that ethical obligations often extend beyond legal and accreditation requirements.

COMMUNITY ROLE

- Health care institutions should be concerned with the overall health status of their communities while continuing to provide direct patient services. They should take a leadership role in enhancing public health and continuity of care in the community by communicating and working with other health care and social agencies to improve the availability and provision of health promotion, education, and patient care services.
- Health care institutions are responsible for fair and effective use of available health care delivery resources to promote access to comprehensive and affordable health care services of high quality. This responsibility extends beyond the resources of the given institution to include efforts to coordinate with other health care organizations and professionals and to share in community solutions for providing care for the medically indigent and others in need of specific health services.
- All health care institutions are responsible for meeting community service obligations which may include special initiatives for care for the poor and uninsured, provision of needed medical or social services, education, and various programs designed to meet the specific needs of their communities.

- Health care institutions, being dependent upon community confidence and support, are accountable to the public, and therefore their communications and disclosure of information and data related to the institution should be clear, accurate, and sufficiently complete to assure that it is not misleading. Such disclosure should be aimed primarily at better public understanding of health issues, the services available to prevent and treat illness, and patient rights and responsibilities relating to health care decisions.
- Advertising may be used to advance the health care organization's goals and objectives and should, in all cases, support the mission of the health care organization. Advertising may be used to educate the public, to report to the community, to increase awareness of available services, to increase support for the organization, and to recruit employees. Health care advertising should be truthful, fair, accurate, complete, and sensitive to the health care needs of the public. False or misleading statements, or statements that might lead the uninformed to draw false conclusions about the health care facility, its competitors, or other health care providers are unacceptable and unethical.†
- As health care institutions operate in an increasingly challenging environment, they should consider the overall welfare of their communities and their own missions in determining their activities, service mixes, and business. Health care organizations should be particularly sensitive to potential conflicts of interests involving individuals or groups associated with the medical staff, governing board, or executive management. Examples of such conflicts include ownership or other financial interests in competing provider organizations or groups contracting with the health care institution.

PATIENT'S CARE

- Health care institutions are responsible for providing each patient with care that is both appropriate and necessary for the patient's condition. Development and maintenance of organized programs for utilization review and quality improvement and of procedures to verify the credentials of physicians and other health professionals are basic to this obligation.
- Health care institutions in conjunction with attending physicians are responsible for assuring reasonable continuity of care and for informing patients of patient care alternatives when acute care is no longer needed.
- Health care institutions should ensure that the health care professionals and organizations with which they are formally or informally affiliated have

†Adapted from the American Hospital Association Management Advisory on Advertising, 1990.

appropriate credentials and/or accreditation and participate in organized programs to assess and assure continuous improvement in quality of care.

- Health care institutions should have policies and practices that assure the patient transfers are medically appropriate and legally permissible. Health care institutions should inform patients of the need for and alternatives to such transfers.

- Health care institutions should have policies and practices that support informed consent for diagnostic and therapeutic procedures and use of advance directives. Policies and practices must respect and promote the patient's responsibility for decision making.

- Health care institutions are responsible for assuring confidentially of patient-specific information. They are responsible for providing safeguards to prevent unauthorized release of information and establishing procedures for authorizing release of data.

- Health care institutions should assure that the psychological, social, spiritual, and physical needs and cultural beliefs and practices of patients and families are respected and should promote employee and medical staff sensitivity to the full range of such needs and practices. The religious and social beliefs and customs of patients should be accommodated whenever possible.

- Health care institutions should have specific mechanisms or procedures to resolve conflicting values and ethical dilemmas as well as complaints and disputes among patients/their families, medical staff, employees, the institution, and the community.

ORGANIZATIONAL CONDUCT

- The policies and practices of health care institutions should respect and support the professional ethical codes‡ and responsibilities of their employees and medical staff members and be sensitive to institutional decisions that employees might interpret as compromising their ability to provide high-quality health care.

- Health care institutions should provide for fair and equitably-administered employee compensation, benefits, and other policies and practices.

- To the extent possible and consistent with the ethical commitments of the institution, health care institutions should accommodate the desires of employees and medical staff to embody religious and/or moral values in their professional activities.

‡For example, the American College of Healthcare Executives' Code of Ethics, and professional codes of nursing, medicine, and so on.

- Health care institutions should have written policies on conflict of interest that apply to officers, governing board members, and medical staff, as well as others who may make or influence decisions for or on behalf of the institution, including contract employees. Particular attention should be given to potential conflicts related to referral sources, vendors, competing health care services, and investments. These policies should recognize that individuals in decision-making or administrative positions often have duality of interests that may not always present conflicts. But they should provide mechanisms for identifying and addressing dualities when they do exist.
- Health care institutions should communicate their mission, values, and priorities to their employees and volunteers, whose patient care and service activities are the most visible embodiment of the institution's ethical commitments and values.

Appendix 2

American Hospital Association

A Patient's Bill of Rights

A Patient's Bill of Rights was first adopted by the American Hospital Association in 1973.

This revision was approved by the AHA Board of Trustees on October 21, 1992.

INTRODUCTION

Effective health care requires collaboration between patients and physicians and other health care professionals. Open and honest communication, respect for personal and professional values, and sensitivity to differences are integral to optimal patient care. As the setting for the provision of health services, hospitals must provide a foundation for understanding and respecting the rights and responsibilities of patients, their families, physicians, and other caregivers. Hospitals must ensure a health care ethic that respects the role of patients in decision making about treatment choices and other aspects of their care. Hospitals

http://www.aha.org/resource/pbillofrights.html (12/12/99). Reprinted with permission of the American Hospital Association, copyright 1992.

must be sensitive to cultural, racial, linguistic, religious, age, gender, and other differences as well as the needs of persons with disabilities.

The American Hospital Association presents A Patient's Bill of Rights with the expectation that it will contribute to more effective patient care and be supported by the hospital on behalf of the institution, its medical staff, employees, and patients. The American Hospital Association encourages health care institutions to tailor this bill of rights to their patient community by translating and/or simplifying the language of this bill of rights as may be necessary to ensure that patients and their families understand their rights and responsibilities.

BILL OF RIGHTS

These rights can be exercised on the patient's behalf by a designated surrogate or proxy decision maker if the patient lacks decision-making capacity, is legally incompetent, or is a minor.

1. The patient has the right to considerate and respectful care.

2. The patient has the right to and is encouraged to obtain from physicians and other direct caregivers relevant, current, and understandable information concerning diagnosis, treatment, and prognosis.

Except in emergencies when the patient lacks decision-making capacity and the need for treatment is urgent, the patient is entitled to the opportunity to discuss and request information related to the specific procedures and/or treatments, the risks involved, the possible length of recuperation, and the medically reasonable alternatives and their accompanying risks and benefits.

Patients have the right to know the identity of physicians, nurses, and others involved in their care, as well as when those involved are students, residents, or other trainees. The patient also has the right to know the immediate and long-term financial implications of treatment choices, insofar as they are known.

3. The patient has the right to make decisions about the plan of care prior to and during the course of treatment and to refuse a recommended treatment or plan of care to the extent permitted by law and hospital policy and to be informed of the medical consequences of this action. In case of such refusal, the patient is entitled to other appropriate care and services that the hospital provides or transfer to another hospital. The hospital should notify patients of any policy that might affect patient choice within the institution.

4. The patient has the right to have an advance directive (such as a living will, health care proxy, or durable power of attorney for health care) concerning treatment or designating a surrogate decision maker with the expectation that the hospital will honor the intent of that directive to the extent permitted by law and hospital policy.

Health care institutions must advise patients of their rights under state law and hospital policy to make informed medical choices, ask if the patient has an advance directive, and include that information in patient records. The patient has the right to timely information about hospital policy that may limit its ability to implement fully a legally valid advance directive.

5. The patient has the right to every consideration of privacy. Case discussion, consultation, examination, and treatment should be conducted so as to protect each patient's privacy.

6. The patient has the right to expect that all communications and records pertaining to his/her care will be treated as confidential by the hospital, except in cases such as suspected abuse and public health hazards when reporting is permitted or required by law. The patient has the right to expect that the hospital will emphasize the confidentiality of this information when it releases it to any other parties entitled to review information in these records.

7. The patient has the right to review the records pertaining to his/her medical care and to have the information explained or interpreted as necessary, except when restricted by law.

8. The patient has the right to expect that, within its capacity and policies, a hospital will make reasonable response to the request of a patient for appropriate and medically indicated care and services. The hospital must provide evaluation, service, and/or referral as indicated by the urgency of the case. When medically appropriate and legally permissible, or when a patient has so requested, a patient may be transferred to another facility. The institution to which the patient is to be transferred must first have accepted the patient for transfer. The patient must also have the benefit of complete information and explanation concerning the need for, risks, benefits, and alternatives to such a transfer.

9. The patient has the right to ask and be informed of the existence of business relationships among the hospital, educational institutions, other health care providers, or payers that may influence the patient's treatment and care.

10. The patient has the right to consent to or decline to participate in proposed research studies or human experimentation affecting care and treatment or requiring direct patient involvement, and to have those studies fully explained prior to consent. A patient who declines to participate in research or experimentation is entitled to the most effective care that the hospital can otherwise provide.

11. The patient has the right to expect reasonable continuity of care when appropriate and to be informed by physicians and other caregivers of available and realistic patient care options when hospital care is no longer appropriate.

12. The patient has the right to be informed of hospital policies and practices that relate to patient care, treatment, and responsibilities. The patient has the right to be informed of available resources for resolving disputes, grievances, and conflicts, such as ethics committees, patient representatives, or other mechanisms available in the institution. The patient has the right to be informed of the hospital's charges for services and available payment methods.

The collaborative nature of health care requires that patients, or their families/surrogates, participate in their care. The effectiveness of care and patient satisfaction with the course of treatment depend, in part, on the patient fulfilling certain responsibilities. Patients are responsible for providing information about past illnesses, hospitalizations, medications, and other matters related to health status. To participate effectively in decision making, patients must be encouraged to take responsibility for requesting additional information or clarification about their health status or treatment when they do not fully understand information and instructions. Patients are also responsible for ensuring that the health care institution has a copy of their written advance directive if they have one. Patients are responsible for informing their physicians and other caregivers if they anticipate problems in following prescribed treatment.

Patients should also be aware of the hospital's obligation to be reasonably efficient and equitable in providing care to other patients and the community. The hospital's rules and regulations are designed to help the hospital meet this obligation. Patients and their families are responsible for making reasonable accommodations to the needs of the hospital, other patients, medical staff, and hospital employees. Patients are responsible for providing necessary information for insurance claims and for working with the hospital to make payment arrangements, when necessary.

A person's health depends on much more than health care services. Patients are responsible for recognizing the impact of their life-style on their personal health.

CONCLUSION

Hospitals have many functions to perform, including the enhancement of health status, health promotion, and the prevention and treatment of injury and disease; the immediate and ongoing care and rehabilitation of patients; the education of health professionals, patients, and the community; and research. All these activities must be conducted with an overriding concern for the values and dignity of patients.

Appendix 3

American College of Healthcare Executives

Code of Ethics

As amended by the Council of Regents at its annual meeting on August 22, 1995. http://www.ache.org/code.html

PREAMBLE

The purpose of the Code of Ethics of the American College of Healthcare Executives is to serve as a guide to conduct for members. It contains standards of ethical behavior for healthcare executives in their professional relationships. These relationships include members of the healthcare executive's organization and other organizations. Also included are patients or others served, colleagues, the community and society as a whole. The Code of Ethics also incorporates standards of ethical behavior governing personal behavior, particularly when that conduct directly relates to the role and identity of the healthcare executive.

The fundamental objectives of the healthcare management profession are to enhance overall quality of life, dignity and well-being of every individual needing healthcare services; and to create a more equitable, accessible, effective and efficient healthcare system.

Healthcare executives have an obligation to act in ways that will merit the trust, confidence and respect of healthcare professionals and the general public. Therefore, healthcare executives should lead lives that embody an exemplary system of values and ethics.

In fulfilling their commitments and obligations to patients or others served, healthcare executives function as moral advocates. Since every management decision affects the health and well-being of both individuals and communities, healthcare executives must carefully evaluate the possible outcomes of their decisions. In organizations that deliver healthcare services, they must work to safeguard and foster the rights, interests and prerogatives of patients or others served. The role of moral advocate requires that healthcare executives speak out and take actions necessary to promote such rights, interests and prerogatives if they are threatened.

I. THE HEALTHCARE EXECUTIVE'S RESPONSIBILITIES TO THE PROFESSION OF HEALTHCARE MANAGEMENT

The healthcare executive shall:

A. Uphold the values, ethics and mission of the healthcare management profession;

B. Conduct all personal and professional activities with honesty, integrity, respect, fairness and good faith in a manner that will reflect well upon the profession;

C. Comply with all laws pertaining to healthcare management in the jurisdictions in which the healthcare executive is located, or conducts professional activities;

D. Maintain competence and proficiency in healthcare management by implementing a personal program of assessment and continuing professional education;

E. Avoid the exploitation of professional relationships for personal gain;

F. Use this Code to further the interests of the profession and not for selfish reasons;

G. Respect professional confidences;

H. Enhance the dignity and image of the healthcare management profession through positive public information programs; and

I. Refrain from participating in any activity that demeans the credibility and dignity of the healthcare management profession.

II. THE HEALTHCARE EXECUTIVE'S RESPONSIBILITIES TO PATIENTS OR OTHERS SERVED, TO THE ORGANIZATION AND TO EMPLOYEES

A. Responsibilities to Patients or Others Served

The healthcare executive shall, within the scope of his or her authority:

1. Work to ensure the existence of a process to evaluate the quality of care or service rendered;
2. Avoid practicing or facilitating discrimination and institute safeguards to prevent discriminatory organizational practices;
3. Work to ensure the existence of a process that will advise patients or others served of the rights, opportunities, responsibilities and risks regarding available healthcare services;
4. Work to provide a process that ensures the autonomy and self-determination of patients or others served; and
5. Work to ensure the existence of procedures that will safe-guard the confidentiality and privacy of patients or others served.

B. Responsibilities to the Organization

The healthcare executive shall, within the scope of his or her authority:

1. Provide healthcare services consistent with available resources and work to ensure the existence of a resource allocation process that considers ethical ramifications;
2. Conduct both competitive and cooperative activities in ways that improve community healthcare services;
3. Lead the organization in the use and improvement of standards of management and sound business practices;
4. Respect the customs and practices of patients or others served, consistent with the organization's philosophy; and
5. Be truthful in all forms of professional and organizational communication, and avoid disseminating information that is false, misleading, or deceptive.

C. Responsibilities to Employees

Healthcare executives have an ethical and professional obligation to employees of the organizations they manage that encompass but are not limited to:

1. Working to create a working environment conducive for underscoring employee ethical conduct and behavior.
2. Working to ensure that individuals may freely express ethical concerns and providing mechanisms for discussing and addressing such concerns.
3. Working to ensure a working environment that is free from harassment, sexual and other; coercion of any kind, especially to perform illegal or unethical acts; and discrimination on the basis of race, creed, color, sex, ethnic origin, age or disability.
4. Working to ensure a working environment that is conducive to proper utilization of employees' skills and abilities.
5. Paying particular attention to the employee's work environment and job safety.
6. Working to establish appropriate grievance and appeals mechanisms.

III. CONFLICTS OF INTEREST

A conflict of interest may be only a matter of degree, but exists when the healthcare executive:

A. Acts to benefit directly or indirectly by using authority or inside information, or allows a friend, relative or associate to benefit from such authority or information.
B. Uses authority or information to make a decision to intentionally affect the organization in an adverse manner.

The healthcare executive shall:

A. Conduct all personal and professional relationships in such a way that all those affected are assured that management decisions are made in the best interests of the organization and the individuals served by it;
B. Disclose to the appropriate authority any direct or indirect financial or personal interests that pose potential or actual conflicts of interest;
C. Accept no gifts or benefits offered with the express or implied expectation of influencing a management decision; and
D. Inform the appropriate authority and other involved parties of potential or actual conflicts of interest related to appointments or elections to boards or committees inside or outside the healthcare executive's organization.

IV. THE HEALTHCARE EXECUTIVE'S RESPONSIBILITIES TO COMMUNITY AND SOCIETY

The healthcare executive shall:

A. Work to identify and meet the healthcare needs of the community;
B. Work to ensure that all people have reasonable access to healthcare services;
C. Participate in public dialogue on healthcare policy issues and advocate solutions that will improve health status and promote quality healthcare;
D. Consider the short-term and long-term impact of management decisions on both the community and on society; and
E. Provide prospective consumers with adequate and accurate information, enabling them to make enlightened judgments and decisions regarding services.

V. THE HEALTHCARE EXECUTIVE'S RESPONSIBILITY TO REPORT VIOLATIONS OF THE CODE

A member of the College who has reasonable grounds to believe that another member has violated this Code has a duty to communicate such facts to the Ethics Committee.

Appendix 4

Model Organizational Code of Conduct

In fulfillment of the organizational goals incorporated in our mission statement and in consideration of the many groups and individuals that have a stake in our organizational activities, the following code of ethical conduct is established as the norm of this hospital.

Governing board members, administrators, staff professionals, employees, associated medical professionals, agents, and anyone else who acts on behalf of this organization shall:

1. Observe strict conformity with all federal, state and local laws, report violations to the compliance officer and request clarification of activities that appear to be out of compliance.
2. Avoid all conflicts of interest and appearances of conflicts of interest in conducting organizational business including strict adherence to organizational rules on gifts and gratuities and on the full disclosure of financial interests.
3. Use only accepted principles and methods of cost reporting and auditing in all financial matters and remain open and fair in resolving disputes.
4. Protect organizational assets from misuse, misappropriation or waste and refrain from using one's organizational position for personal gain.

5. Provide all medically appropriate health care services insuring that no one in need of care to stabilize his or her medical condition will be turned away and that no one will be discharged without a plan that will safeguard his or her welfare.

6. Provide health services in accordance medical ethics standards and with patient self-determination as stated in the Patients' Bill of Rights giving special care to the interests of patients who are in vulnerable conditions or who are participating in medical research.

7. Be sensitive to the social, cultural and religious needs of patients and their families, giving special care in respect to requests for organ donation.

8. Maintain the confidentiality of patient information and proprietary information of the organization.

9. Be honest and fair in marketing and promotional presentations and in media relations.

10. Conduct governmental relations and personal political activities in such a way as to reflect the mission goals and ethical principles of the institution.

11. Treat patients, employees and associates with respect and without discrimination regardless of age, race, religion, gender disability, ethnicity, political affiliation, or sexual orientation.

12. Adhere to the standards of one's own profession.

Appendix 5

American Hospital Association Policies and Positions (Excerpts)

Community Accountability with Changes in the Ownership or Control of Hospitals or Health Systems

PREAMBLE

Communities are facing many changes in their health system, including changes in its ownership and control. In all cases, the reason for and the outcome of these changes should better serve the sick and improve the health of the community through a more efficient and effective health system.

PRINCIPLES FOR CHANGES IN OWNERSHIP OR CONTROL

Hospitals and health systems are important resources for their communities. When planning a change in ownership or control, hospital leaders should educate and inform their communities—including medical staff and employees—in a timely manner of the objectives for the change, the process being followed, and the opportunities for community comment.

The core values of a hospital or health system are defined by its mission, including emphasis on its role of caring for the sick and improving community health. Board decisions with regard to changes of ownership or control should be made within the mission of caring for the sick and improving community health.

GUIDELINES FOR HOSPITAL/HEALTH SYSTEM LEADERS WHEN CHANGING OWNERSHIP OR CONTROL

Boards are encouraged to adopt these guidelines as policy for their institution/ system before considering any proposal to change ownership or control.

- Work with the community to identify its health needs and the resources that are available to improve the health of the community and to meet its needs for health services. Ensure there is a plan for the provision of care to the under-served in the community as well as the continuation of other essential community services.
- Identify your organization's values and goals in advance of considering an ownership change. Adopt criteria for evaluating any change in ownership or control before examining proposals.
- Encourage compatibility in values and philosophy by favoring changes that reflect shared missions, visions, and strategies. Develop a communication plan that involves and informs all constituencies, including medical staff and employees.
- Obtain a valuation, by a party not involved in the transaction, of charitable assets being converted or restructured to ensure receipt of reasonable value is received or used in structuring the transaction.
- Identify financial incentives which may influence the views of trustees and executives involved in proposing and evaluating any change in ownership or control. Disclose all conflicts of interest, offers of future employment, future remuneration, or other benefits related to the transaction.
- Control and administer any foundation or charitable trust created by the transaction separate and distinct from the restructured health care organization.
- Ensure that a foundation, charitable trust, or community payment created from transaction continues to serve an appropriate health need charitable purpose of the community.
- Disclose publicly the terms of an agreement to transfer control or ownership once a letter of intent (or memorandum of understanding) is signed. Provide an opportunity for public comment on the transaction before it is final.

- Inform the appropriate state official, usually the attorney general, of the terms of a transaction once a letter of intent (or memorandum of understanding) is signed.

Appendix 6

Joint Commission on Accreditation of Healthcare Organizations

Sample Components of an Organization Ethics Framework

- Organization mission, vision, philosophy and values statements
- Publication or distribution of ethics standards and mission and values statements to the community
- Mechanisms for receiving and using public feedback about the ethical performance of the organization
- Use of community members on governing bodies and advisory committees with explicit mandate to monitor the ethics of the organization
- Conflict-of-interest policies for the governing body, senior managers, and staff
- Corporate compliance plan for fraud and abuse prevention and monitoring
- Financial management, reimbursement, and billing policies and practices
- Human resource management policies for staff selection, promotion, confidentiality of employee information such as salary and health status, transfer, disciplinary action, harassment, benefits, and termination
- Policies rewarding exemplary ethical behavior in the organization, as well as handling violations discreetly and respectfully

Source: Joint Commission, *Ethical Issues and Patient Rights Across the Continuum of Care*, Oakbrook Terrace, IL: Joint Commission on Accreditation of Healthcare Organizations, 1998 page 74. Reprinted with permission.

- Policies addressing the ethical use of financial incentives for managers, physicians, and staff while ensuring integrity in clinical decision making
- Accurate marketing representation of the organization's scope of services, hours of service, fees, admission criteria, and relationships with other organizations
- Discharge planning practices, especially if the patient is referred to another service of the organization
- Referral relationships with other organizations of practitioners
- Relationships with vendors
- Policies governing admissions and the transfer of patients to other organizations
- Policies on acceptance of gifts or cash
- Information management policies which protect patient confidentiality
- Codes of conduct addressing personal and professional boundaries between patients and staff
- Policies on solicitation of donations from patients, families, vendors, and the community
- Administrative policies and organization practices which ensure compliance with applicable law and regulation
- Strategic planning initiatives that consider community needs and just resource allocation
- Grievance mechanisms
- Institutional Review Board (IRB) policies and procedures
- Partnership and joint venture agreements
- Marketing and advertising plans
- Policies governing the relationship of the organization to affiliated organizations, including educational institutions

Index

DATE DUE

	OCT 15 2009		